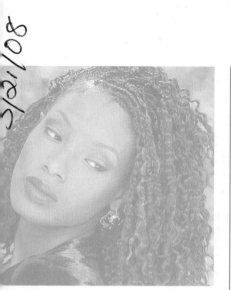

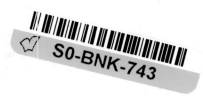

The World of Wigs, Weaves, and Extensions

Toni Love

MILADY

THOMSON LEARNING

Australia Canada Mexico Singapore Spain United Kingdom United States

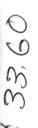

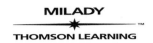

MILADY

THOMSON LEARNING

The World of Wigs, Weaves, and Extensions
by Toni Love

MILADY STAFF

President:
Susan L. Simpfenderfer

Publisher:
Marlene McHugh Pratt

Acquisitions Editor:
Paul Drougas

Developmental Editor:
Patricia Gillivan

Editorial Assistant:
Rebecca McCarthy

Executive Production Manager:
Wendy A. Troeger

Executive Marketing Manager:
Donna J. Lewis

Channel Manager:
Wendy E. Mapstone

NOTICE TO THE READER

Dedication

This book is dedicated to my mother, who saw the gift in me that I did not see. You have always kept your hands in the small of my back, and your sweet voice remains in my ear, saying, "You can do it. You can do anything you want to do." This is one of many motivating tools you have passed to me. To my deceased father, I miss you every day. To the remainder of my family, I love you.

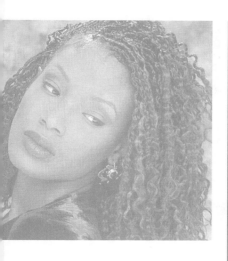

Contents

CONTENTS

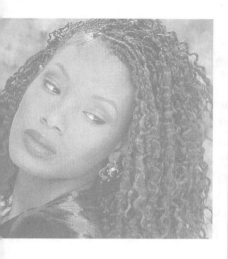

Foreword

Since recorded history, human beings have used various techniques to simulate hair. Throughout humankind's existence, social orders have used the wig for fashion and ceremony. Archeologists have recorded this phenomenon in social structures all over the world, in every race and culture. Among the artifacts and wall paintings of ancient Egyptian tombs and excavations are an abundance of wigs and hairpieces. These artifacts tell of the pieces' daily uses. The image of Cleopatra would be incomplete without the striking geometric lines of her bangs and the straight ends of the bobbed wig in which Cleopatra is commonly depicted.

While modern technology has produced an enormous number of synthetic fibers that simulate natural hair, the art of creating wigs and using hair substitutes was a highly developed craft before modern science. Early craftspeople used henna and other products to dye hair. Fashionable male and female nobles of the Roman empire were known to use wigs and hairpieces. Often these nobles cut the hair of their blond slaves to add exciting new colors to the predominantly dark hair colors of the Italian peninsula. The Romans may have adopted this practice from the Greeks, whom the Romans conquered and from whom much of Roman society evolved. Like many other peoples, Romans may have started wig use for the theatre or opera.

Because human hair, like gold, sugar, tobacco, and other commodities, has always been valued by the world's societies, it is conceivable that hair was among the merchandise Marco Polo brought back from China. Italy remains one of the great human-hair processors and is considered the finest in the world by many knowledgeable members of the extensive international hair trade.

Europe sustained brisk wig manufacturing and trade that lasted for hundreds of years, well into the 19th century. Among the vast number and variety of notable historical figures who used wigs were poets, generals, kings, queens, and statesmen. There is abundant historical reference to wig use by Thomas Jefferson, George Washington, Queen Elizabeth of England, Louis the Fourteenth and, the most famous wig-wearer, Marie Antoinette. Members of the British court still wear wigs today.

Currently, all hair comes from the Orient. This includes such synthetic fibers as konekolon, which was developed and rose to popularity during the middle of the 20th century. It is in the Orient that new developments have imitated and refined textures. One such development simulated African American textures in wigs and hairpieces. Sales of human and synthetic hair have made the industry one of the major international markets today, in the billions of dollars.

Africa's contribution to the sale and art of hair and hair-replacement fibers is evident in many areas of pop culture. African Americans were probably the first to seek materials to use as hair. The most popular of these is "African Lent." A tremendous variety of braids, twists, and dreadlocks were developed in Africa and brought to the Americas by the African Americans who settled in the New World. Hair is one of the few African arts that has survived the transition to the Western Hemisphere, commonly used by most people in North, South, and Central Americas, as well as the Caribbean. In many cases, hair is a cottage industry that is integral to African American culture.

Each era in the exciting history of wigs has provided craft innovations and never-ending opportunities for hair designers. Contemporary cosmetologists can and do enjoy this highly lucrative area of hair design via the tremendous developments in processing and materials. Specialists may realize enormous profits from expertise in wigs, hairpieces, and the currently popular hair extensions. Training is an essential part of the cosmetologist's repertoire.

This book defines the latest wig and hairpiece technology and presents technical understanding of the subject. This book includes information from some of the most informed sources available, among them Toni Love. Written by a dedicated instructor and knowledgeable artist with extensive experience in every facet of cosmetology, this book is a viable tool and should be revered for its factual information on the subject of wigs, hairpieces, and hair extensions.

Torain

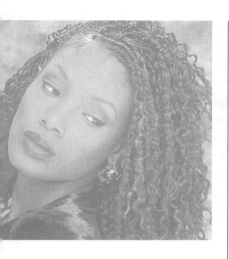

Acknowledgments

First, I would like to thank Torain, the "Fusion Master," for answering my letter and inviting me to my first international hair show. Thank you for reaching back and helping me. I'll never forget you. I would also like to thank Susan Simpfenderfer for giving me the opportunity to pursue my dream of writing this book. To Pam Lappies, thank you for always staying positive, making me feel comfortable, believing in me, and introducing me to Paul Drougas. Thank you, Paul Drougas, for encouraging me, taking chances on me, and giving me this opportunity. Thank you, George, for the support, love, and understanding you provided while I worked on this project. Thank you, Willie Braggs, for sharing your ideas with me and continuing to offer your support. A special thanks to my only brother, Les, for being there when I encountered "computer jams" and for offering his love and support. I would also like to thank my students; my clients, especially Georgia; my church family; my Greensboro community; my co-workers, especially Pam; and my friends, especially Shirley, who believed in me. Finally, thank you all for your prayers and words of encouragement. May God bless all of you.

The following people were instrumental in my development as a professional: Superintendent Miles; Superintendent Joseph Dantzler; Mr. J. J. Purter; Mrs. Rhinnie Scott; Mrs. Purter; Mr. Spiver Gordon; Mr. Dedrick Hodges; Mr. and Mrs. Hank Sanders; Mr. Robert Turner; Mr. Joe Dudley, President of Dudley Products, who helped change my life; Mr. and Mrs. Gary Marlow; Mrs. Pamela Anderson-Cole, who is still a very dear friend; Mrs. Pam Strong, who always offered words of encouragement; Mrs. Beth Englebert; Mrs. Jeanene Collins, who always offered funny and kind words; Mrs. Patrice Johnson-Thomas, who always helped with enrollment; Mrs. Shirley Johnson, who was always honest and encouraging; Mr. Ed Winslow; Ms. Betty Brown; Mrs. Janice Hendrix; Mrs. Shirley Spencer; Mr. Lorenzo Freeman; the custodial staff who have always helped in any way they could (you know who you are); my former and current students Lakeisha Duke, Lanasia Bell, Tyrone Madison, Ferell Moss, Loretta Bozeman, Tracy Washington, Cindy Acker, Jimmy Maddox, Latoya Simmons, Bobbie Conner, Tiffany Hobson, and many others; Mrs. Debbie Hammonds, who helped me finish this book by being patient, consistent, and encouraging; Edith Abakarae, Rita Watts, Debra Buckman, Claude Beson, Susan Walker, Barbara Powell, and other members of the staff at Sally's Beauty Company; Mr. Hayford and Mrs. Davis of Stillman College; Dr. Wilkerson and Dr. Green-Burns of the University of West Alabama; Dr. Theodore Dixie of Alabama A & M University; and Victor Poole and the staff of the Bank of Melville. Thanks again!

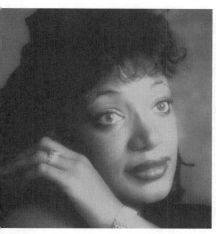

About the Author

Toni Love is a native of Greensboro, Alabama. She attended Greensboro Public School, West Campus, and joined the United States Army Reserves while in high school. After completing basic and advanced training, she attended a private cosmetology school, Hair Design Academy, where she was instructed by Walter and Jo Boyd. Toni attended Stillman College and the University of Alabama and received a Bachelor's degree in Business Administration concentrating in Business Management. She received a master's degree in Continuing Education from the University of West Alabama and is pursuing an Educational Specialist degree in Career and Technical Education from Alabama A & M University.

Toni comes from a family of beauty professionals—her mother is a beautician and her uncle is a barber—and Toni began working in her mother's salon when she was 14 years old. Today, Toni is the Director of Continuing Education for Dudley Products. She has written another book entitled *Tips to Pass the Cosmetology State Board Exam,* and she has created a Web site, http://www.tonilove.com.

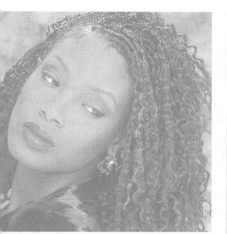

CHAPTER 1

Why Wear a Wig?

There is no one reason people wear wigs. Over the years, wigs have been used in almost every capacity. As we embark on the era of holistic healing, wigs have more to do than with just looks. Wigs can be associated with the individual's soul and mind. In early times, wigs protected the scalp from the sun. Early politicians and clergy members wore wigs. Members of the high courts were known for their hairstyles, many of which were white wigs with curls on both sides.

Deciding to Change

Before attempting to wear wigs, people must first be honest with themselves and understand the aspects of changing hairstyles, as well as the reasons they are seeking to change their hairstyles. Before changing their hairstyles to wigs, people should ask themselves questions like, "Is this a temporary change or a permanent change?" "Is this a medical change or a fashion change?" "Is this change prompted by a self-esteem issue?" "Am I seeking a change because everyone else is doing the same?" For a person who has undergone chemotherapy that has resulted in hair loss, for example, the change to a wig is more than a fashion trend. All clients must get in touch with their souls and be truthful as to their desires and their options.

Once people have established why they are seeking a hairstyle change, the transition to wigs is easy. As a next step, clients should learn their hairstyle options and decide which options are best for them. Stylists and doctors cannot make these decisions for clients, but emotionally distressed clients, such as burn patients, clients with bad cases of alopecia, and clients who have lost hair due to thinning or breakage, may seek answers from these professionals. Clients like these need attention because they are under a lot of stress. Few clients do their own research and therefore depend on their stylists to have all the answers about hair care and hair-care options. Not every stylist knows all the facts of hair care and wig selection, however. It takes a gifted, compassionate, and patient stylist to serve stressed clients.

The bottom line in these situations is that hair exerts psychological effects from the past, present, and future. The past represents the time when clients had their own hair and could change their hair if they wanted. The present is the situation clients face now, which is hair loss. Sudden hair loss is more detrimental to the client than hair loss due to thinning and breakage, which are more gradual. Clients usually take action when hair loss due to thinning or breakage becomes noticeable, sometimes hurrying to find answers to their hairstyle and hair-care questions. The future is the time during which clients must make sure they are comfortable with their decisions and the answers they have received.

Making the Change

Today, men and women alike are working more than ever before. Therefore, the average worker is under a lot of stress and has or takes little time for hair maintenance. As a result, there is a lot of hair loss due to neglect, and there is a growing demand for the convenience of wigs and weaves. In a family with parents who are working and children who are involved in extracurricular activities, there is little or no time to sit and enjoy a home-cooked, healthy dinner. When a poor diet is paired with the stress of the everyday routine, hair loss results.

Versatility is another reason people wear wigs or weaves. Approximately half the women in the United States are fashion conscious. A lot of women will change their hair at least three to four times a month. African American women alone spend billions of dollars on their hair. Men are just as conscious of hair loss as women, if not more, so wigs and weaves are also prevalent among men. Hair-loss and hair-replacement products and treatments that are geared to the male population are advertised all the time. The toupee has been around for years to help men with their hair-loss problems. There has long been color on the market to help men "fill in" their thin areas, and there have been wigs throughout the years for men. Men today spend millions of dollars on hair-loss cosmetics, hairpieces, toupees, and full wigs.

The severe damage resulting from the use of harsh chemicals can cause clients to seek hairstyle options. Few people understand the seriousness of chemical damage. Some people color their hair at home, while others go to salons for color applications, but color is a chemical. If the basic principles of color are not fully understood, a person can have serious problems. If, for example, a woman colors her hair and decides the next day to again change her color, the damaging process begins. If a week later the woman decides to color yet again, the damage is in full effect. As time progresses, the hair weakens and starts to shed. A person may begin to feel stress, another damaging factor. If the woman in this example had other chemicals in her hair, such as a relaxer or a permanent wave, she could have major and possibly sudden hair loss. To avoid this possibility, the woman could wear a wig of the desired color until deciding to change her color permanently.

In addition to color, wigs can be worn to give the hair a rest from such chemicals as relaxers, permanent waves, soft curls, and texturizers.

Wigs can also be worn for flexibility and durability. In an interview with Barbara Walters, Diana Ross said she " . . . wore wigs because they were easy to deal with during traveling." Wigs can be seen on such modern celebrities as Lil' Kim, Christina Aguilera, Mary J. Blige, and Tina Turner. Wigs and weaves are so prevalent today that many people are tempted to try one, but people should get in tune with themselves before attempting this new look. Once people get in tune with themselves and know who they are, they can wear wigs or weaves with such an attitude that other people would be afraid to ask, "Is that your hair?" Instead, people will say, "I love the new you!"

Embracing the Change

Consider a student who suffers from A-Topic Dermatitis, a skin disease she inherited from her father and for which she has been taking medication since age 2. The student's hair grew long until a relative, who did not consider the then-preteen student's skin disease, decided to apply a soft-curl permanent to the student's hair for easier maintenance. The student's hair came out in clumps and did not grow long. The result was permanent hair loss. Today, approximately 6 years later, the student's hair is the same length.

About 4 years ago, the student finally decided to try a wig. Her father had suggested a wig for years. She must wear wigs made of 100 percent human hair because of her skin disease. Today, the student, now a young mother, is proud that she decided to try a wig. She stated in a recent interview that she feels much better about herself, that her self-esteem is at an all-time high, that she has started to take better care of herself, and that she has started wearing makeup to enhance her new look. The student feels that wearing a wig has changed her life and has given her a sense of pride she had only dreamed of, as well as the motivation to go on with her life.

Another woman, a retired schoolteacher, had an experience one could only imagine. On a warm day this woman was pulling figs from a tree when she was attacked by ticks. The severity of the attack and the amount of venom secreted by the ticks caused the woman to suffer severe hair loss and skin problems. She stayed in shock for some time after the incident. After a while, with the support of family and friends, the woman decided to seek answers to her hair and skin problems. She started with a dermatologist, then moved to her hairstylist. The stylist suggested treatments for the woman's almost bald scalp, as well as a weave, but the woman was afraid of the weave's bonding glue and had too little hair for another method. She had consulted with her doctor before receiving the scalp treatments. As an option, the woman bought a wig and went to a stylist who specializes in hair enhancements. That visit restarted the woman's life, and the wig made a tremendous difference in the woman's appearance.

The woman wore her wig until her hair grew back to its natural length and in an interview stated that she will continue to wear the wig because she likes having choices. In fact, the woman has purchased several other wigs to try different styles and colors. For this retired school-teacher, a wig was an option during a time of distress, but choosing to wear one was difficult. When she did make that decision, however, she found a new look and a new outlook on life. Like the young student, the woman regained self-esteem and self-assurance.

In yet another case, a middle-aged, recently divorced adminis-trator wanted a new look. She decided to start with her hair and bought a wig. At first, the woman felt insecure, asking such questions as, "What if it slides off?", "What is everyone going to say?", "What if it is too thick and bushy?", and "What if it's the wrong color?" After she wore the wig for a few days without incident, the woman realized that the wig was a positive change. Co-workers and fellow church members said things like, "What have you done? You look so good!", "I like the new look!", and "Divorce has been good to you." These comments gave the woman the fuel she needed to experiment even more. She started buying wigs with streaks and highlights to enhance her looks, and now the wigs have become such a part of her life, she never wears her natural hair out in public.

As mentioned earlier, people wear wigs in the entertainment business. Female singers who travel a lot wear wigs for versatility. Males in the entertainment business use wigs to promote their characters and their acts. Comedian Flip Wilson, for example, dressed as a female on his show using wigs and makeup. Jamie Foxx did the same with his character "Wanda" during the *In Living Color* television series, as did

Martin Lawrence with his character "Sha Na Na" on the television show *Martin*. Other males, like RuPaul, have made cross-dressing part of their entertainment personae and are rarely seen out of character. Wigs are also important to people who enter pageants and perform in musicals and shows.

Wigs are worn by anyone who needs or wants them. There are no requirements as to who can wear a wig or how old a person has to be to wear a wig. Children can be stricken with such conditions as cancer, dermatitis, alopecia, and burns and at young ages suffer hair loss. Children can be cruel, and children with conditions like these can be sensitive. Parents should be aware of the psychological effect of hair loss on children. In cases like these, children have choices, too: wigs. Wigs can be made specially for children's small heads. A salon in Manhattan invited women to have their hair cut and donated for children's wigs. The children were grateful for the women's hair, which when sewn into wigs was styled with ribbons for a youthful look.

Like they do for adults, wigs help children look and feel good. Children with hair loss may seem distant or quiet due to low self-esteem. They may perform poorly in school because they will not ask questions that may draw attention to themselves. They may not display their talents because they do not feel good about themselves. Whether the hair loss has an internal or an external cause, parents should remember their children's cosmetics.

Children's hair loss can stress parents as well as children. Parents can be so focused on reassuring their children that they do not explore all options. Some parents may feel that a child is too young for a wig and let the child instead wear a cap that is offered to most medical patients. Children may still want hair, whatever the option, especially if they had hair before. Therefore, parents should include their child in the decision-making process. When children are included in decisions, they begin to recover, because they can start to feel hopeful. Also, their self-esteem can begin to rise.

Whatever the wearer's age, the question remains: "Why wear a wig?" There is no one answer. The answer may have nothing to do with hair loss, style or fashion, or the latest fad. The wig wearer may be a housewife, a doctor, a lawyer, a teacher, or a 6-year-old child. It does not matter why clients wear wigs, and it does not matter who wears wigs. The answer to the question lies in each individual.

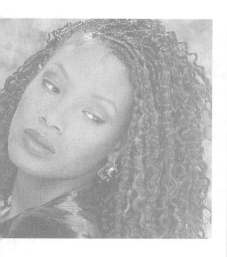

CHAPTER 2

Types of Wigs

Once people decide to wear wigs, they should research the types of wigs that are best for their needs.

Hand-Tied Wigs

One type of wig is the hand-tied wig (Figures 2–1 and 2–2). This wig is expensive, because each hair is sewn individually to the base of the wig. This wig is made of 100 percent human hair, which gives the wig a natural look. The hand-tied wig must be cleaned with a special fluid that must be used with extreme care.

Some wigs are hand-tied around the hairline to give the client a natural look. Hair can be attached in any design to the crown of this wig, which means that the crown will meet the needs of the client and will give the client unlimited performance and satisfaction. This type of wig can be requested from a wig-manufacturing company.

Machine-Made Wigs

Another type of wig is the machine-made wig (Figures 2–3 through 2–5). Machine-made wigs are cheaper than hand-tied wigs. Wefts, which are strips of material to which hair is sewn, are sewn

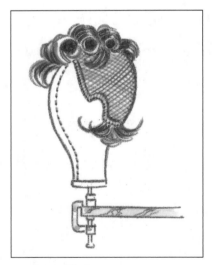

FIGURE 2–1
Hand-knotted wig.

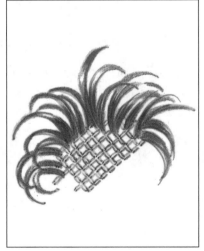

FIGURE 2–2
Hair crocheted and hand knotted into mesh foundation.

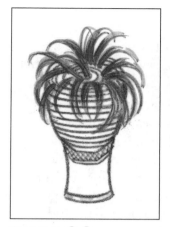

FIGURE 2-3
Weft wig (top view).

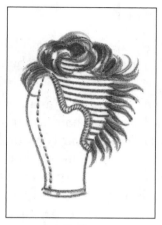

FIGURE 2-4
Weft wig (side view).

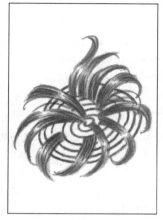

FIGURE 2-5
Hair sewn by machine into net cap or weft in circular rows.

together onto a mesh cap to create machine-made wigs. The wefting of machine-made wigs creates wigs that are spaced correctly for proper balance and distribution. These wigs are not too thick or too thin. These wigs cover the head and give the head balance. Clients who wear machine-made wigs will not have to worry that their wigs are too long on one side or too short on the other. In machine-made wigs, the hair is commonly triple-stitched to the webbing or to the mesh cap with transparent thread to extend the wigs' durability. Elastic adjustment bands in the back of these wigs help fit the wigs and make them comfortable.

Machine-made wigs differ from hand-tied wigs in that machine-made wigs tend to be more bulky and more difficult to style. Machine-made wigs can be more difficult to style because their hair is sewn at certain angles or in certain directions or patterns. Clients who want to style their wigs differently or comb their wigs in different directions may have problems. For example, if the hair in a machine-made wig is sewn downward but the client wants the hair combed upward, the client may have a problem getting the hair smooth. If the wig hair is long, the ends may turn upward nicely while the hair closest to the scalp may not cooperate as well. Hand-tied wigs, with their hair stitched individually, give clients more styling versatility.

Making Wigs from Hair

When selecting wigs, clients must find hair textures that match their own hair textures. When they do, their changes are not drastic; they are more transitional.

Wigs can be made of European human hair, which is the most expensive type of wig hair. European hair, which is easy to work with, ranges from dark to light. European hair is natural looking for people who have this hair texture and who want to change hairstyles without cutting or adding such chemicals as permanent waves or color. Asian hair, which is straight and dark, is another kind of hair that can make up wigs. This hair, which seems plentiful, is cheaper than European hair, and is coarse.

Indian hair is relatively cheap, usually limp, and dark. As a result, Indian hair is not the most popular in the industry. However, this hair is real, tends to give wigs a natural look, and some feel it is easy to work with. One disadvantage of this hair is that, once it is collected, it has to be sorted by length and color, a process some companies feel is difficult and time consuming.

Hair produced by horses and sheep, the latter called angora, is used more in hairpieces than in wigs. Hairpieces made of animal hair are often used for models in hair shows and hair competitions. Animal hair is soft and fine and usually has a glasslike finish. Hair produced by yak, a type of ox found in Asia, has become popular in the hair industry. Yak hair is considered one of the best types of hair among consumers. It gives the hair a somewhat coarse look and tends to be popular among African American consumers. This hair is natural looking when mixed with angora. Yak hair in wigs is best when mixed equally with angora. It gives the wig natural effects, and the hair tends to style better. The other advantages of yak hair are that it is cheap and plentiful. Therefore, most consumers can obtain the hair for usage.

Synthetic hair is also used for making wigs (Figure 2–6). Synthetic hair is manufactured from several fibers, including nylon, dynel, and acetate. Synthetic wigs are inexpensive and plentiful. Wigs made of synthetic fiber can be used every day, but clients must take special precautions. For example, a client wearing a synthetic wig must prevent too much heat from contacting the wig, because the wig will

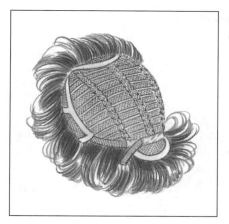

FIGURE 2–6
Synthetic, handmade stretch wig.

singe where exposed to heat. Heat from an oven or a too-hot curling iron will singe the wig.

Half-Wigs

Last, there are half-wigs. Clients who want to add hair to the backs of their heads use half-wigs. The hair on half-wigs is usually the same length as the hair on full wigs. Half-wigs are used to add thickness and body to newly created styles, and they are used to enhance natural hair, because natural hair is left out in some areas when styling. Half-wigs can be used to create styles or to fill in thin spots, and they can be used to add length to short sides.

Half-wigs are made on a round, ventilated, flat base with metal clips on two sides to secure them. Half-wigs offer the versatility of full wigs, but at a more modest price. In addition, they are plentiful and come in different textures, styles, and colors. Securing and blending half-wigs require a special touch. The half-wig must be placed carefully where the client wants or needs it most, because once the wig is secured and the hair is styled, the wig must be resecured and restyled if the client does not like the result. When the styling requires molding with styling gels and setting lotions as well as drying time, this procedure can be time-consuming. In most cases, however, half-wigs are practical and easy to use daily. For clients going through gradual hair loss or clients

11

interested in nondrastic changes, half-wigs may be an option before graduating to full wigs.

Choosing a Wig

Because there are many types of wigs on the market today, clients can have any look they want. Clients must decide which wigs are best for them. All clients cannot wear the same wig. A student with dermatitis, for example, can only wear wigs made of 100 percent human hair to prevent irritation and other problems. Clients must know that synthetic wig fiber is flammable.

The kind of hair in wigs is important to all clients. Match tests can identify a wig's type. This test helps to determine if a wig is made of man-made fiber or human or animal hair. To conduct this test, burn a small amount of the wig's hair. Synthetic hair melts and beads at the end. The hair will feel burned or singed, and there is usually no odor during burning, though a slight odor is emitted after burning. Human hair has a strong, sulfurlike odor during burning.

Wig selection is important to men as well as women. The most common wig for men is the toupee, which is often used to cover baldness on the top of the head. The hair on the sides of the head is usually blended with the toupee for style purposes. Toupee application may be less tedious than wig application, because the toupee is secured with an adhesive.

Toupees, like wigs, come in different types. Male clients must be informed about their options. Store owners or workers should be able to provide helpful information about the wigs they are retailing, but if they cannot, clients must read wig labels themselves. Hairstylists consulting on wigs on the market should make sure to be aware of all a client's medical conditions and allergies. Wigs can be constructed of fibers as well as colors; therefore, client consultation is important in selecting the best wig for a client's needs.

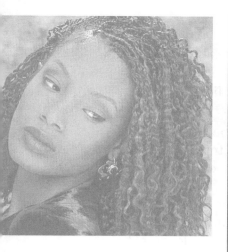

CHAPTER 3

Wig Measuring and Ordering

When clients decide to wear wigs, they submit to consultations during which stylists complete record cards of the clients' hair history and medical history. The stylist helps the client choose an appropriate wig according to the client's information.

Measuring the Client

Before measuring and ordering any wig, the stylist should ensure that the client wants to wear a wig. It is important that the stylist avoids appearing overbearing. Instead, the stylist should let the client lead the decision-making process.

To measure a client for a wig, start by encircling the client's head with measuring tape, from the nape of the neck, over the top of the ears, and along the front edge of the hairline (Figure 3–1). To measure accurately, write down the measurements, then measure again. Next, measure the client's head from front to back by placing the tape at the hairline in the center of the forehead, over the crown to the center of the hairline at the nape of the neck (Figure 3–2). Again, write down the measurements and repeat for accuracy. Then, measure across the client's crown from the top of one ear and over the crown to the top of the opposite ear (Figure 3–3). Write down the measurements and repeat for accuracy.

There are six procedures for accurately measuring clients for wigs:

1. Around the head—Measure from the nape to one ear, to the front hairline, to the other ear, and back to the nape.
2. Width of the nape—Measure from behind one ear to the nape, to behind the other ear (Figure 3–4).
3. Front center—Measure from the hairline to the center bottom of the nape.

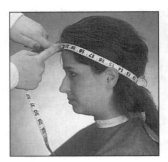

FIGURE 3–1
Measure the circumference of the head.

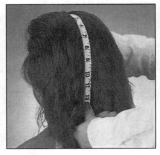

FIGURE 3–2
Measure from the hairline at the middle of the forehead to the nape.

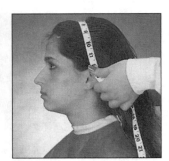

FIGURE 3–3
Measure the top of the head.

4. Sideburn to sideburn—Measure directly over the head.
5. Ear to ear—Measure over the forehead (Figure 3–5).
6. Sideburn to sideburn—Measure directly across the occipital bone (Figure 3–6).

When measuring clients for toupees, note the circumference of the head. The most important measurement is the area the toupee will cover. Use a water-based marker to mark the client's head where the toupee will end in the front and on the sides. If the client's bald or thin area is on the top of the head and joins the crown, measure that area. If there is hair on the sides of the client's head, consult with the client as to how far into that hair to blend the toupee.

Once the wig or toupee is measured properly and accurately, the client is ready to make other, cosmetic-related decisions before ordering the wig or toupee. A few of these cosmetic decisions involve hair color, texture, and type. Clients must decide if their wigs will be in their natural hair color or another color. Clients must decide if straight, curly, kinky, or wiry hair is desired. Stylists should have hair samples of all types to show clients before ordering so clients will know what to expect. Pictures are helpful as well, but the opportunity to touch hair while looking at a picture of someone wearing the hairstyle helps reassure the client.

The stylist should contact wig manufacturers to obtain various hair samples. From the beginning of the consultation process preceding wig ordering, it is important for the client to know wig prices. Some wigs

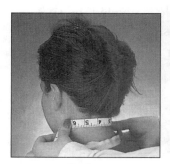

FIGURE 3–4
Measure the width of the nape line.

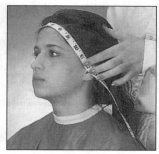

FIGURE 3–5
Measure across the forehead.

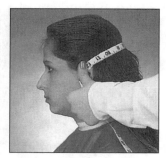

FIGURE 3–6
Measure from temple to temple.

are affordable, some are expensive. However, a wig that may be less expensive may be low maintenance but less durable. Therefore, a client with such a wig may have to order frequently. A wig that is more expensive may give the client the feel of natural hair and may be more durable. The more expensive wig should be of better quality and give the client more styling versatility. Toupees are somewhat more expensive than wigs. When toupees arrive, the stylist or barber will call the client in for a "try-on," at which time the stylist or barber may need to make some adjustments. For example, the barber may need to cut and style the toupee to blend with the hair on the sides of the client's head, or the stylist may need to color the client's hair to match the toupee. The manufacturer may require a hair sample be sent with the order to ensure color accuracy.

The client who wears a toupee every day may need to order a second before the first wears out from such events as constant combing and brushing. Some clients like to try to shampoo and style their toupees but may cause problems doing so. The adhesive may not stick as well after a certain period, or the hair in the toupee may start to thin. If any problems occur, it is time to order another toupee or another wig. Wigs will eventually lose their luster and shine, styles will start to lose their shape, and the hair will start to thin. When a wig starts to lose its shape and the hair starts to thin, it is time to order a new wig. If wig luster fails to enhance a wig's style, it is time to order another wig. When ordering a second or even a third wig, stylists should be sure to take clients' measurements again to ensure accuracy. The stylist should also again consult with the client to be aware of special problems, any medical conditions, and any changes. If another hair sample is needed, be sure that the hair is clean and is the color the client desires. The stylist should keep a record card on every client and send a copy to the wig manufacturer, wig supply store, or wig dealer.

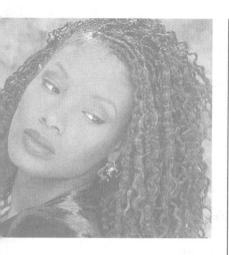

CHAPTER 4

Blocking and Fitting the Wig

The wig block holds or secures the wig for styling when the wig is not being worn. The block is also used during fitting and when the wig needs cleaning. Wig blocks are commonly made of canvas and styrofoam, although they are also made of other materials, and they come in different sizes. Some wig blocks have colored covers; some are white with no added color.

The different sizes of wig blocks should be considered, because wigs can stretch. If a wig has been ordered to fit a client's head securely and the client has a wig block that is substantially larger than the client's head, the wig will likely stretch and become too loose for the client.

Securing Wigs to Wig Blocks

Wigs are secured to wig blocks with wig pins, commonly called T-pins. These pins, which are shaped like the letter *T*, are thin and have pointed edges like needles. To secure the wig to the wig block, carefully place T-pins through the wig hair and cap (Figures 4–1 and 4–2). Wig or T-pins help eliminate sliding and falling. They also help maintain the wig's style. The client can secure the styled wig on the wig block for wearing the next day. Styrofoam blocks can be used to demonstrate pinning and styling the wig, and they can be used in wig stores to display wigs. Styrofoam blocks are less expensive than wig blocks and can be ordered by the dozen or the case for a very reasonable price. For the client who wears several different wigs, the styrofoam block is ideal for securing and storing wigs. Wig block clamps can also be used with wigs and wig blocks.

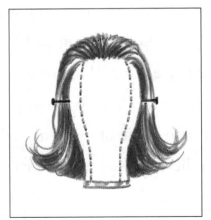

FIGURE 4–1
Place one T-pin at the center of the forehead and one at each side.

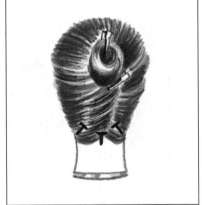

FIGURE 4–2
Place one T-pin at the center of the nape and one at each corner.

Fitting Wigs to Clients

For a client with a small head, the stylist may have to shrink a wig. To shrink a wig, the wig base or cap must be moistened, placed on a small wig block, and allowed to dry naturally. To maximize accuracy of the fit, the stylist should measure the client's head and wig block again.

Clients with large heads may have difficulty finding wigs that fit. For these clients, the stylist may have to stretch wigs. To stretch a wig, moisten the wig base or cap and place it on a large wig block. Secure the wig with T-pins and allow it to dry naturally. Again, the stylist should measure the client's head and the wig block to ensure accuracy in fit.

Wigs with adjustable bands in the back help secure the wigs to clients' heads (Figure 4–3). Some clients like the bands, others do not. Some clients with small heads have knotted the bands to keep their wigs from sliding. Wigs come with combs as well as bands. The combs are placed in the client's natural hair near the scalp to secure the wig. Wig clients with thick hair tend to prefer combs over bands because wigs fit more snugly and securely with combs. Clients have danced, done aerobic exercises, and lived full lives with wigs with comb attachments. Bald clients cannot wear wigs with combs, however, because some natural hair is needed for the combs to attach.

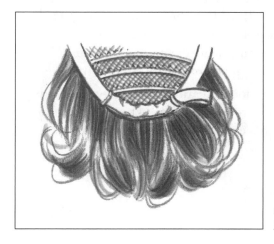

FIGURE 4–3
Elastic band.

19

Ensuring the Fit

To help the client ensure that the wig fits, the stylist should comb the client's hair back and pin it down. Carefully holding the wig side flaps and elastic band to the back, the stylist should then place the wig over the client's forehead and lower it over the client's head. With one hand applying pressure at the front of the client's head, the stylist should hold the wig in place. With the other hand at the back of the client's head, the stylist should stretch the elastic band over the pinned hair, being careful to protect the styling of the wig. When the wig is in place, the stylist should make small adjustments in the styling of the wig with the fingers, a teasing comb, a styling comb, or a brush. If the wig feels insecure, the stylist should insert one or two bobby pins in the netting on both sides, in the top close to the client's forehead, or in the client's nape area. The bobby pins should be the same color as the hair on the wig so as to avoid bringing unnecessary attention to them.

Helping the Client

Once the wig has been properly cleaned and styled on the block, it is ready to wear. The stylist should make time during the consultation to teach the client about properly fitting and removing the wig. If the client has problems, the stylist should repeat the procedure and allow the client to practice fitting and adjusting the wig. The stylist should conduct the client consultation privately and afford the client ample time to ask questions before leaving with the wig. It is always a good idea to do a follow-up consult with the client after a few weeks to ensure client satisfaction. Some clients require special attention and follow-up calls.

Once clients understand wig blocking and fitting, they are ready to learn how to clean and make minor repairs to wigs. They may need these skills if they cannot afford to have them done professionally.

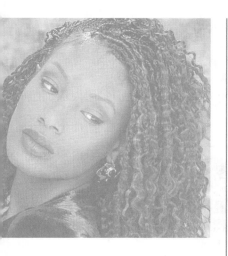

CHAPTER **5**

Cleaning and Repairing the Wig

Wig cleaning depends on the number of times the wig is worn and the wig's hair type. For example, if a wig is made of human hair and is worn daily, the client should clean it every 2 weeks. Wigs can accumulate a buildup of hairsprays, hair sheens, wig luster, and the oils that are used to enhance wig appearance. Smoke and other fumes can cause a wig to have an unpleasant odor. Human-hair wigs are more absorbent of odors than synthetic wigs.

Wigs should not be shampooed in extremely hot water. Always follow the manufacturer's instructions for cleaning the wig. The wig block is useful when cleaning the wig, because it secures the wig with the help of T-pins (Figures 5–1 and 5–2). When the wig is secure, brush out the hairspray and any other dirt and residues that have accumulated on the wig.

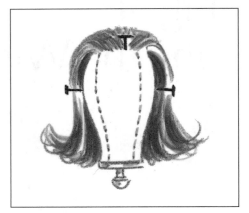

FIGURE 5–1
Front view.

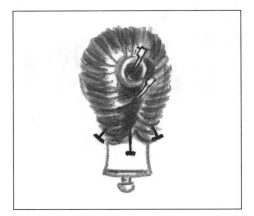

FIGURE 5–2
Back view.

Taking the Right Steps in Cleaning

Use gloves when cleaning the wig to protect the hands, because some wigs must be cleaned with a special nonflammable cleaner (Figure 5–3). A glass basin is also suggested for wig cleaning. Before immersing the wig in the solution, follow the manufacturer's directions as to the amount of wig cleaner to place in the basin. Once the wig is in the basin, make sure it is saturated with solution. Dip the wig in and out of the solution several times, making sure the wig does not tangle (Figure 5–4). When finished cleaning, squeeze the wig gently, lay it on a towel, and pat it dry (Figure 5–5). The wig can then be placed back on the wig block, secured with T-pins, and left to dry. Once the wig is dry, it is ready to be conditioned (Figure 5–6). The wig can also be conditioned in a glass basin, if needed. If the area closest to the head, which is the cap, needs more cleaning, use a Q-Tip™ to access that area.

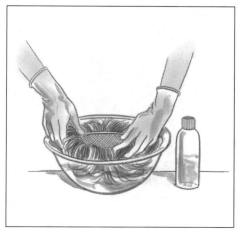

FIGURE 5–3
Wash the wig with a nonflammable liquid cleanser.

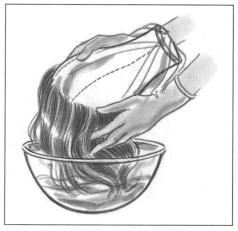

FIGURE 5–4
Saturate the wig and work the solution through the hair.

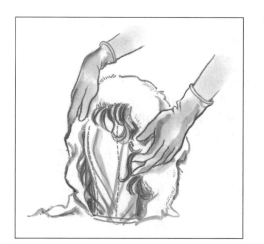

FIGURE 5–5
Towel-dry the hair.

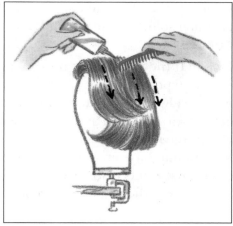

FIGURE 5–6
Condition the wig after cleaning.

If the wig block is made of a material that cannot sustain water or moisture, the client should cover the block with a plastic cap or Saran Wrap™ for protection (Figure 5–7). The wet wig can be placed on the protected surface and secured for drying and styling (Figure 5–8). When rinsing the wig, make sure that the water is cool or tepid, and rinse the

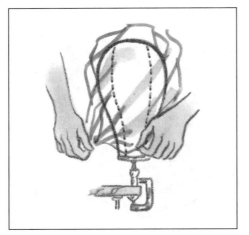

FIGURE 5-7
Covering the block.

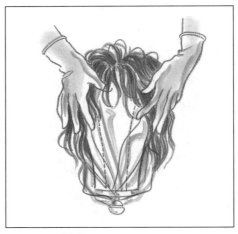

FIGURE 5-8
Placing the wig on the block.

wig more than once to ensure that it is free of cleaning solution. If cleaning solution remains in the wig, the skin and scalp may become irritated.

If the wig is curly or wavy in texture, whether it is a synthetic or a human type, the client should make sure not to brush or comb the wig excessively, because excessive combing or brushing will disturb the wig's curl or wave pattern and the wig will no longer look the way it did when it was purchased. The client who brushes or combs excessively will likely have to purchase another wig to recapture the original style. If the wave or curl pattern is disturbed, and the client chooses not to purchase another wig, the wig may be repaired.

Repairing the Wig

Wig repair is not difficult, but the client should allow the stylist the opportunity to repair the wig. The stylist or wig specialist is a professional who has trained in such technical skill areas as hair cutting, hair shaping, hair sculpting, and hair molding. A wig that may seem damaged and distorted to the client may just need a new cut or a new style. A wig can look new after simple deep conditioning with the appropriate conditioner. The conditioning of wigs depends largely on the type of wig and the type of hair from which the wig is made. A client who does not know this may do more damage to the wig than good. When clients disturb the natural curl or wave patterns of their wigs, they can try to change the style of their wigs by rolling and restyling the wigs. A stylist or wig specialist can offer restyling suggestions.

Wig repair can be as simple as cutting off the ends of the hair on the wig, because when a wig is worn regularly or for a long period, the ends may start to look shabby or uneven. The repair of a synthetic wig may include clipping off the singed ends of the wig instead of replacing the wig. The bands on the wig can be replaced or tightened to avoid replacing the wig. Combs on wigs may need to be glued back into place. A client, a stylist, or a wig specialist can make these minor repairs to a wig.

Clients must understand that when wigs are taken to salons and left for cleaning or repair, the stylist or wig specialist will charge for the services. When clients choose to leave their wigs for services, they should be sure to ask and answer all questions. When a wig is severely damaged, the stylist or wig specialist may have to spend extra time or more time than scheduled to repair the wig. Repair costs depend on geographic area. Some clients visit cosmetology schools to get their hair and their wigs worked on by students. The students gain experience and clients cut costs. Before seeking wig repairs this way, however, clients should speak with a cosmetology instructor to find out if the students are learning wig care. After the wig has been repaired, if it will not be worn immediately a wig case for storage is a wise investment. The wig case is designed to store the wig during travel and at home. A wig case provides the protection a fine wig deserves.

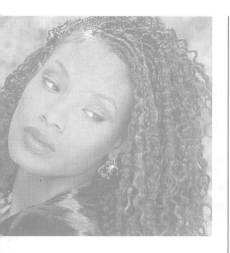

CHAPTER 6

Shaping and Styling the Wig

As stated in Chapter 5, a wig may need cutting or clipping for repair reasons, or the client may just desire a new style. In any situation, "hair shaping" or hair cutting, as many call the technique, is irreversible. Hair cannot be reattached to the wig. Therefore, it is important that the client take the wig to a stylist or wig specialist who is trained in wig hair shaping or hair cutting.

Cutting Wig Hair

Wigs may be cut with hair-cutting shears, thinning shears, clippers, or a razor. When the wig hair is cut with hair-cutting shears, the wig hair can be wet or dry. If the wig is too bulky for the client and must be thinned, the wig hair must be dry. Clippers can be used on wet or dry wig hair, but dry hair yields the best results. A razor is used on a wig when the wig hair is wet or damp.

There are several hair cuts for wigs. The basic layered cut is the most practical for the client who desires no particular style. If the wig is purchased with no definite pattern, the basic layered cut can give the client more styling choices.

Cutting the Basic Layered Cut

The procedure for a basic layered cut with shears or clippers is as follows:

1. Section the hair into four or five sections (Figures 6–1, 6–2, and 6–3). (If the client wants bangs, section the hair into five sections to ensure a definite bang area.)
2. In the nape area, find the guideline by taking smaller sections of hair from the large sections. Use the comb to measure the

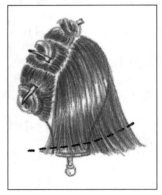

FIGURE 6–1
Part a 2 inch (5 cm) guide-line and cut to the desired length.

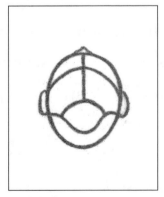

FIGURE 6–2
Top front.

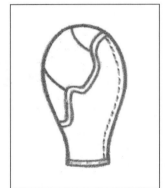

FIGURE 6–3
Right side.

length desired by the client. (The guideline in the nape area is the guideline around the perimeter of the head.)

3. Cut around the perimeter of the head, using the guideline in the nape area (Figures 6–4, 6–5, and 6–6). (This cut is the same as the blunt cut. A blunt cut is cutting the hair using a stationary guideline and holding the hair straight up, down, or out at a 90° angle.)

4. Part the hair down the middle of the head and divide the hair into two large panels. Pin one whole side so that it does not interfere with cutting on the opposite side. Hold the hair straight up in a 90° angle and start cutting in the front of the head, laying down hair that is cut and picking up uncut hair. Proceed to the back of the head. Repeat this step throughout the top of the head. When the sides are reached, pull the sides straight out toward you and cut. (There will be little hair to cut from the sides, because most was taken off during the blunt cut.)

5. Once the unpinned side of the wig is cut, pin this side and repeat Step 4 on the other side. At the conclusion of this step, the whole wig should be cut from front to back. To check for accuracy and even ends, make small parts from side to side, holding the hair up in a 90° angle, and cut as needed. Once the wig has been cut and checked, it is ready for styling.

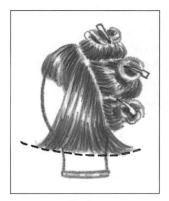

FIGURE 6–4
Left side of the head. This illustrates a completely cut guideline.

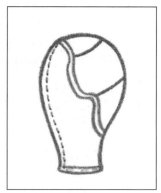

FIGURE 6–5
Left side.

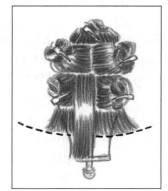

FIGURE 6–6
Back of the head. Let down center back hair. Cut to the same length as the guideline.

The procedure for the basic layered cut can be done with clippers or shears or both. If both implements are used, make sure the client understands that each implement achieves a different effect. During the consultation, the stylist or wig specialist should always explain to the client the effects of the implements to ensure client satisfaction.

Thinning Wig Hair

If the wig has a lot of hair and the client wants to keep the hair long, the stylist or wig specialist should suggest thinning the wig. Thinning takes little time and removes bulk and excess hair without removing length. There is no particular procedure for thinning a wig. The stylist or wig specialist should consult with the client as to the specific wig areas to be thinned. If the client wants the wig thinned all over, the stylist or wig specialist should follow the procedure for a basic layered cut (see preceding section) but take small sections and thin close to the ends of the hair, not close to the scalp. When hair is thinned too close to the scalp, the hair tends to stick up or to cause overlapping hair to stick up.

Cutting Wigs with Razors

For best results when cutting with a razor, make sure the wig hair is wet or damp. Like thinning, there is no particular procedure for cutting with a razor, but when unsure, follow the procedure for a basic layered cut (see preceding section). With a razor, cut the hair closer to the ends than to the scalp. A razor gives a lot of different effects to the wig in different areas. Therefore, it is imperative that the stylist consults with the client before attempting to cut the wig with a razor. A few cuts and effects to achieve with the razor are:

- Long graduation cut
- Short graduation cut
- Layered cut
- Twist cut
- Wisping
- Slithering
- Blocking
- Tapering
- Blending

Completing the Razor-Cutting Procedure. The following cutting technique is commonly practiced on wigs when using the razor:

1. Stand slightly to the side. Section the hair from the center of the forehead to the center of the nape.
2. If a bang effect is desired (the bang area is the first section), taper the first section with the razor.
3. With the razor flat on top of the second section (slightly behind the bang area), taper an inch away from the scalp area or wig cap, down the hair shaft. Cut to the desired length. Continue to the crown area and the center of the temple.
4. Take a side section, approximately 2½″ back, and, holding the hair straight downward, cut. This is the guideline for the front. (This technique is called "blocking.")
5. Go back and taper as needed, blending the top area and the sides. Continue to taper the hair until the center back is reached. Once the center back is reached, use it as a guideline for continuing to the other side of the head.
6. Continue the cut from the back to the front, or start the cut from the front and go to the center back, where it will need to be even with the opposite side. Be sure to hold the razor very flat to taper evenly without hair stubs.
7. Direct the hair forward from the crown and cut even with the front section to achieve a double length or layered look in the crown area.

There are many razors on the market. Therefore, stylists and wig specialists should make sure to be familiar with the hair type of wigs to be cut with razors. Some of the hair may be coarse; some may be fine. These factors impact which effects the razor gives the wig. It is also important that clients understand what razors can and cannot do to wigs. Clients who bring their wigs in for razor cutting should stay until their wigs are finished so that they know what is done and why.

Getting a Good Wig Cut

A good hair cut is the foundation of a good hairstyle, whether the hair is cut with a razor, haircutting shears, or clippers or it is thinned with thinning shears. A record card should be kept on each client of the procedure performed on the wig and the procedure results. The record card should also include which implements were used on the wig to achieve the results, and any special procedures or precautions or client desires. The record card should be kept in an active file, because the client may call at any time inquiring about hair-cutting or hairstyling procedures or products. A client may come in with another wig and ask the stylist or wig specialist for a cut completed on a previous wig. If this happens, the stylist or wig specialist can pull the client's record card and follow its notes of instruction.

Styling the Wig

The principles of modern hairstyling are basic guides in selecting which wig styles are most appropriate and which will achieve the best results. The wig style should emphasize the client's best features and minimize the client's poor features. In modern hairstyling, the best results are achieved when facial and head shapes are analyzed. Each type of face requires a distinctive hair design that is proportioned, balanced, and designed to frame the face.

The hairstylist or wig specialist must have basic knowledge of hairstyling and wig styling and a sense of balance and harmony to keep up with the demands of hairstyles and wig styles. The skilled and successful stylist or wig specialist gives each style personal flair so that the style is personal and attractive and suits the individual.

The essentials of artistic and appropriate wig styling are:

- The shape of the head—Front view, side view (profile), back view, and type of hair on the wig
- Personal characteristics—Best features (emphasize and use as the foundation of styling), imperfect features (minimize), defects and blemishes (conceal)
- Body structure and posture

In considering these general characteristics, the stylist or wig specialist is afforded the opportunity to visualize the hairstyle or wig style desired for the client, and the stylist or wig specialist can plan appropriate hair-cutting techniques. The client should realize that a good hairstyle or wig style is not only becoming and in fashion, but easy and quick to handle. The hair should be styled to permit the client to easily groom and maintain the hair.

Identifying Facial Shapes

Several facial shapes must be considered when designing a wig style or hairstyle for a client:

- Oval—Usually considered the perfect facial proportion. This face is about 1½ times longer than it is wide across the brow; the forehead is slightly wider than the chin. The styling objective is to maintain the oval contour. Any hairstyle can be worn, depending on the client's preference.
- Round—Contours usually give a circular impression. This face is wide across the eyes and cheeks with a short, rounded chin line. The styling objective is to create the illusion of length. When styling, the hair can be cut shorter and styled wide at the top of the head and lifted for height and balance. The nape area can be styled close to the head.
- Square—Features are usually especially wide across the forehead, cheekbones, and jaw line. The styling objective is to create the illusion of length and to offset the squareness of the features. When styling, the ears can be concealed and the nape area can be kept long and full, with the hair reaching below the line of the jaw or the chin.
- Triangular—Features a narrow forehead, a wide jaw and chin line, and a large or thick neck. The styling objective is to create the illusion of height and width across the forehead. The hair should be styled close to the head to conceal the ears and longer in the nape and close to the neck.
- Rectangular or oblong—Features are usually narrow and long. The face appears long and the cheekbones appear sharp. The styling objective is to make the face appear shorter and wider. The hair should be styled fairly close to the top of the head and forehead. The hair should be partially draped to combine with fullness at the sides to help reduce the apparent length of the face.

- Diamond shaped—Has a narrow forehead, wide cheekbones, and a narrow chin line. The styling objective is to create the illusion of less width across the cheekbone line. The layered cut is suggested for this facial type, with full bangs falling on the forehead. The hair is usually kept full and wide in the back and nape areas.
- Thin—Usually characterized by a narrow forehead, a pointed chin, and hollow cheeks. The styling objective is to transform the facial shape. The hair should be left long and shaped smooth in the nape area and smooth but wide on top.
- Narrow and bony—Appears narrow and thin. The styling objective is to create an illusion of youth. The hairstyle should be long and full.

Making Special Considerations

When creating wig styles for clients, it is important for the hairstylist or wig specialist to consider back views. In fact, the stylist or wig specialist should make sure that the style looks good from all views. The stylist or wig specialist should not allow the client to leave the salon or shop with straggly, unshaped, or disorderly hair, which means the stylist must consider the client's neck. Clients with short necks should wear their hair short in the nape area but high on top. In contrast, clients with long necks should leave their hair long in the nape and back.

When styling hair or a wig for a client, the stylist or wig specialist should also consider the client's profile. There are four common profiles:

- Straight—Client usually has good features and harmonious contours. Nearly all hairstyles are becoming.
- Concave—Appears on clients with bulging foreheads and strong or massive lower jaw lines. The hairstyle or wig style should minimize these features. The layered cut is suggested for this client. Bring the hair forward from the crown and leave it full behind the ears.
- Sharp angular—Appears on clients with full chins and receding foreheads. The top of the head is narrow. The styling objective is to disguise these contours. The receding forehead and pro-truding chin can be corrected with a hairstyle or the correct

wig style. The hair should be styled forward on top to fall half-draped across the forehead.

- Convex—Indicated by a receding forehead, protruding nose, and receding chin. The styling objective is to minimize these features. The hairstyle or wig style should have bangs to fall over the forehead. The layered cut is suitable for this client, and the hairstyle should be full with height and volume.

Once the stylist has consulted with the client and considered the client's facial shape, profile, and neckline, the stylist should gather and sterilize all necessary implements before starting to style. In addition, the stylist or wig specialist should prepare the workstation. A prepared and organized workstation is very important. Once the area is prepared, the stylist or wig specialist can be available for any client who walks through the door. Following are some implements that may be needed for styling wigs:

All-purpose comb	Hairspray	Wave clamps
Tail comb	Hair spritz	Towels
Teasing comb	Oil sheen	Styling capes
Handle comb	Curl wax	Neck strips
Bristle brush	Permanent wave rods	Shears
Wire paddle brush	End papers	Clippers
Vent brush	Hair nets	Razor
Magnetic rollers	Single-prong clips	Thinning shears
Thermal curling irons	Double-prong clips	Heater
(electric/marcel)	Duckbill clips	Wig block
Blow-dryer	Hair pins	T-pins
Setting lotions	Bobby pins	
Mousse	Roller pins	

Combs come in various shapes, lengths, and sizes, so it helps the stylist or wig specialist to know the advantages of each type. It is important that the stylist or wig specialist hold combs correctly when rendering services to clients and ensure proper balance and control at all times. It is also important for the stylist or wig specialist to hold shears correctly and to work with shears of the proper size. The stylist or wig specialist should "palm" the shears to maintain control of the shears and to protect the client.

Roller size is important when styling a wig. Roller diameter plays an important role in the size of curl the client receives during styling. The longer the hair on the wig, the larger the roller must be when styling. When rollers are placed in a wig for setting, the rollers may be on-base to produce strong lift or strong curl effect. The base is the area where the hair strand extends from the scalp. The rollers may be half-base to give the hair volume. The rollers may be off-base to give closeness and direction to the nape or along the hairline. When a stylist or wig specialist lacks rollers or the client simply desires volume, barrel curls can be used instead of rollers. Barrel curls roll the hair like rollers in a manual procedure that gives the wig hair maximum volume. Like roller size, wig texture is important in achieving proper styling results. The size of the client's head and the length of the wig hair are important attributes in roller placements. Human-hair wigs yield better results when using rollers to set the hair (Figures 6–7 through 6–10).

Wave clamp, styling clip, bobby pin, hair pin, and roller pin functions depend solely on the needs of the stylist or wig specialist. Pins can be used to secure pin curls as well as rollers. Hair pins and bobby pins can be used to secure French twists, French rolls, and any other "up-do" styles. Because hair pins, bobby pins, wave clamps, and roller pins are available in various sizes, they can be used on short as well as long wigs. Single-prong and double-prong clips can be used to secure shaping. Wave clamps can be used to secure waves that are placed in the

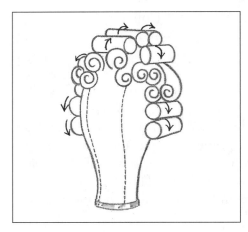

FIGURE 6-7
Setting on block.

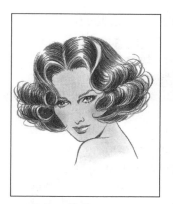

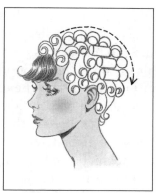

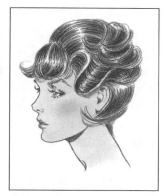

FIGURE 6–8
Finished style.

FIGURE 6–9
How the setting would look on the head.

FIGURE 6–10
Finished style.

wig for styling purposes. Hairsprays have different functions with wigs and hair in general. Some hairsprays are designed to hold the hair in place; some apply fragrances. Some wig lusters apply shine and gloss to a wig; others help set wigs in style. Because there are many different sprays on the market with many different uses, it is important to read labels. Some sprays may work well on natural hair but not on synthetic fibers. Some sprays may be gummy and damage the wig. Because wigs come in so many textures, it is important for clients to learn as much home wig maintenance as possible.

Long wigs can become matted and tangled during shampoo and reconditioning. Before water is applied to the wig or after the wig is shampooed, it is important to remove all tangles. The stylist or wig specialist should do so by always starting in the lowest part of the nape area. Small parts should be made to keep the sections thin and free of excessive pulling and breaking. The hair should be combed from the ends of the strands toward the scalp area. The stylist or wig specialist should comb the tangles from the hair very gently. The stylist should proceed this way through the wig, making small parts until the wig is tangle free.

Clients may request that some type of part be added to their wigs to achieve a particular style. If stylists or wig specialists are unsure about where to place the part, they should comb the hair back from the hairline using a large-tooth comb. Then, using the index finger in the area the client requested, they should direct the comb beside the index finger, starting at the front hairline. Next, the stylist should comb at the top of the index finger and separate the hair at this point. Then the stylist should comb the crown hair in an upward motion and the opposite hair in a downward motion, continuing to comb the crown hair upward, away from the new part. The stylist should be sure not to extend the part too far back into the crown area. The hairline on the wig as well as the growth pattern of the wig must be considered. Hair does not grow on wigs. Therefore, the pattern in which the hair was sewn into the wig or hand-tied to the wig plays an important role in making parts. Many wigs have parts when purchased. When this is the case, the established part may be difficult to remove.

When selecting a wig style, clients should not try to imitate other people. A hairstyle will look different on everybody. It is not that hair trends are not important. Celebrities and musicians have always set hair and fashion trends; they give the general public new and intriguing looks. However, stylists and wig specialists have a duty to be honest with their clients. They should tell their clients when styles are unbecoming and give clients the resources to explore other options before allowing those clients to select inappropriate wig styles.

To maintain a wig in a way that is suitable for the client, the client is obligated to keep the wig:

- Clean, because the hair will be more manageable
- Cut and shaped regularly, if the wig is going to be worn regularly
- Styled appropriately and serviced according to its needs

If clients incorporate these elements into their "wig lifestyles," then home maintenance will be problem free.

Identifying Wigs

Wigs come in various styles with various names, depending on the manufacturing company. Over the years, there have been several names for wigs based on their styles, such as "the flip." The flip consists of a smooth crown, a casual bang, and hair ends flipped upward. This wig style was popular among young women. The "French twist" wig style consists of gentle curls and soft movement with the hair twisted upward in the back. This style was worn during the day, but it was also worn at night for an evening of elegance. The "beehive" is another wig style that was once popular. This style consists of a smooth base and high drama in the crown area. This wig style can be worn with a bang and hair hanging elegantly around the sides, somewhat straight, or somewhat curly, whichever the client prefers.

Wig styles have changed considerably throughout the years. This is evident when looking back on the days of such wig-wearing entertainers as The Supremes, Tina Turner, and Billie Holiday. During the 1950s and 1960s, the hottest singing group or actress influenced hairstyles. Today, this remains true. The public watches entertainers for trend-setting hairstyles and fashions. Professional wig styling can achieve some styles.

Knowing the type of wig is helpful in this regard, because the hair type tells the wig stylist what can and cannot be done to the wig. For example, if the wig is made of synthetic fiber, the stylist knows that an abundant amount of heat cannot be used on the wig. If the wig is made of human hair, the wig can be curled with curling irons, roller set, and set on permanent rods for a curly look.

Wig hair can be pin-curled to achieve curly looks, as well. Banana clips and scarves can aid in styling the wig. If the client chooses to use the banana clip in the wig hair, the client should make sure that the wig has a moderate amount of hair, because once the hair is pulled upward with the clip, the mesh wig cap should not be visible. Some wigs have attached headbands for styling purposes. If a wig has an attached headband, it has styling versatility. The wig can be pulled toward the back of the head for a half-wig look, as if the client has a ponytail. For the days the client does not want to expose any natural hair, the client can wear the wig with headband leaving the hair around the hairline exposed.

Wigs can be styled with setting lotions, sculpting gels, mousses, pomades, and dry fast. Dry fast is a light, liquid solution sometimes used to dry the hair of roller sets, fingerwaves, and various wet sets. The wig hair can be roller set into desired styles with these styling aids. For example, the "Lolita" wig style can be achieved by:

1. Pin-curling the nape area and rolling the back area downward with medium or larger rollers.
2. Rolling the top backward, rolling the bang area forward, and pin-curling the sides above the ear toward the face.
3. Drying and styling the wig.

The "flip" is achieved by:

1. Allowing the bang area to hang loosely.
2. Rolling the nape area and sides upward.
3. Rolling the top and the crown toward the back with large rollers.
4. Rolling the temple areas on both sides downward.
5. Drying and styling the wig.

The "wrap" is achieved by:

1. Taking a wig with straight hair that is lacking body on the ends and dividing it into four sections: Section 1 is the right back crown, Section 2 is the left back crown, Section 3 is the front left side, and Section 4 is the front right side.
2. Once the hair is divided properly, make sure it is saturated with wrapping lotion.
3. Start to comb Section 1 into Section 2, Section 2 into Section 3, Section 3 into Section 4, Section 4 into Section 1 until the hair is wrapped into a circle with a smooth crown.
4. Thoroughly dry and comb out the wig the way it was wrapped, starting with Section 1.

The drying time for this style may be longer than expected, because the hair overlaps. A properly wrapped wig style results in a lot of body on wig hair ends. Results are best on human-hair wigs or wigs made of yak.

Other popular wig styles are the:

- Short layered pixie—Short and lightweight wig that gives the client a classic look.
- Page Boy—Mid-length wig that is bluntly cut with a soft bang.
- "Crimpy waves"—Short-cut wig with crimpy-looking waves that is tapered close to the sides and to the back of the head.

- Microbraids—Wig that is braided in microbraids and cut into a short-cropped style. This is one of the most popular wig styles of the early 21st century.
- "Dreadlocks"—Wig that gives the "Rasta" look of the Caribbean Islands. The hair can have a rough or a smooth finish.
- "Spiked"—Wig with a spiked cut with the look of a razor finish. The hair stands throughout the top of the head and gives a look of excitement.
- "Wet Look"—Wig that is dry but so glossy it looks wet. This wig comes in a layered cut or a blunt cut. The hair comes straight or in Jherri curls.
- "Curly Perm"—Wig that can allow the client the versatility of curls without the permanent wave process.
- "Wispy Braids"—Wig that has braids that are not as small as microbraids. The braid ends are loose, and the wig hair is cut so that the ends are wispy in the bang and nape areas.
- "Shag"—Wig that is short in the front and longer in the back. The "shag" style is a "comeback" from the 1980s.
- "Spring Curls"—Wig full of tiny spring curls that gives the client a carefree look. This style is popular among clients who desire a natural look.
- "Feather Cut"—Wig that is feathered and has a tapered back to give the client a look of elegance. This wig offers the client softness.
- "Wet and Wavy"—Wig that has a wet look and a wavy style. This style offers a carefree look that allows the client to look relaxed.
- "Spiral Curls"—Wig that gives the client the look of a spiral perm wrap without the permanent wave process.
- Relaxed bob—Wig that is cut in a bob style. The hair is soft and shiny, silky straight, and gives the client the look of a new relaxer without the process of chemical relaxing.
- "Corkscrew"—Wig that is made of corkscrew hair and is cut close to the nape area and full in the top area.
- "Kinky Bob"—Wig that has a "kinky" look. This wig is for clients who have no desire for chemicals but want to experience a change.

- "Headband"—Wig that is suited to the active client. A head-band attached to the wig provides extra security. This wig comes in all colors, styles, and hair textures.

Short-style wigs are known to sometimes give a sense of softness. These wigs are a little less maintenance than other wigs, but they do require a lot of rolling. The short-style wig can be wrapped to give some body. Short-style wigs made of human hair can be shampooed, blow-dried, and thermal-curled. Short-style wigs made of synthetic fibers need little, if any, thermal curling. Synthetic wigs usually hold their style a little longer than human-hair wigs. Weather changes affect human-hair wigs, which require a little more attention than synthetic-hair wigs. Most short-style wigs can be brushed gently and sculpted into style.

Short-style human-hair wigs can be rolled on small rollers if longer-lasting curls are desired. Rollers yield longer-lasting curls than do curling irons. This is true with long human-hair wigs, short human-hair wigs, and wigs made of yak hair.

Wig styles today are eclectic. Shopping for a wig is almost like shopping for clothes or shoes, there are so many choices. Wig styles range from curly, to wavy, to straight, to braids, to finger waves, to wet and wavy styles, to dreadlocks. In the wig arena, there is something for almost everybody. Once a client decides to wear a wig, styling it is as easy as styling natural hair. However, the client must become familiar enough with the wig to know what is right for the wig and what is wrong for the wig. With this information, styling is easy. If clients are ever in doubt about the styling of their wigs, though, they should always consult a professional.

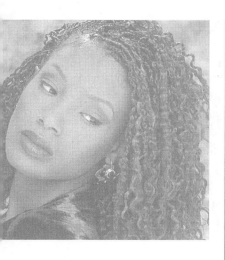

CHAPTER 7

Wig Coloring

Hair color is categorized three ways: permanent, semipermanent, and temporary.

Differentiating Hair Colors

Permanent color lasts until it is cut out, grows out, or is colored over. Permanent colors require peroxide for their color development. The peroxide comes in 10 volume, 20 volume, 30 volume, and 40 volume. The volume helps indicate the strength and processing time of the color. For example, color mixed with 10 volume peroxide undergoes slow processing. Color mixed with 40 volume processes faster. Clients should not engage in wig coloring, because doing so can be tricky. They should take the wig to a wig specialist or to a professional stylist. If clients choose not to consult a professional, they must ensure that they have a great deal of knowledge and experience with regard to wig coloring.

Semipermanent color lasts from 4 to 6 weeks and fades from shampoo to shampoo. This color will not change the texture of the hair on the wig, but it will change it temporarily. The client should understand that semipermanent color is most effective when clients want darker hair. Some clients who want lighter hair for short periods do not realize that semipermanent color will not give them the desired effect.

Temporary colors, which are the same as color rinses, last from shampoo to shampoo. They are only beneficial when clients want darker wigs. Temporary colors do not lighten wig hair, although color rinses can be purchased in lighter shades for clients with those hair or wig colors. If clients desire light wigs, they may consider shopping for wigs in light shades.

Whether color is permanent, semipermanent, or temporary, the client must always follow the manufacturer's directions for proper application. If not, the client may have a major disaster, something like wig hair that is too light or too dark, a change in wig hair texture, or uneven wig hair color. Wig hair is usually colored with the wig on a canvas or styrofoam block. Be sure to protect the canvas or styrofoam block with a plastic cap or Saran Wrap. When the client is unsure of color results, a strand test on the wig is wise. Take the strand of wig hair from an area of the wig that will not be noticeable. Most strand test hairs are taken from the nape area. To conduct the test, place the strand of hair in an appropriate amount of aluminum foil and mix the color according to the manufacturer's directions. Apply the color to the strand of hair and leave it on for the required time. A spray bottle can be used to rinse the hair, then towel-dry and blow-dry the hair to see the color. If there is still doubt about the color, take the wig outside, after the strand is dried, and view the color.

Coloring a Wig/Hairpiece

Following is the procedure for coloring a wig/hairpiece.

1. Ensure that the wig/hairpiece is clean.
2. Pin the wig/hairpiece to the canvas or styrofoam block.
3. Select the color and apply it to the wig/hairpiece thoroughly and rapidly. Be sure to pay close attention to the time and the manufacturer's directions. In most cases, the wig/hairpiece will receive hair color quickly. If using color with peroxide, apply it only to dry hair. Because peroxide is known to destroy or deteriorate the foundation of the wig or hairpiece, be careful not to saturate the foundation with the color. Take strand tests every 5 minutes to ensure satisfactory results (Figure 7–1).
4. After the appropriate processing time, rinse the wig/hairpiece thoroughly.
5. Shampoo the wig/hairpiece thoroughly according to the manufacturer's direction, and rinse.
6. Apply a cream rinse/conditioner to the wig/hairpiece.
7. Comb the hairpiece into the desired style and dry (Figures 7–2 and 7–3).

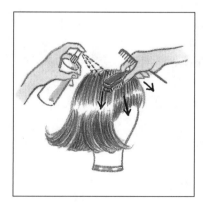

FIGURE 7–1
Spray the hair with color rinse.

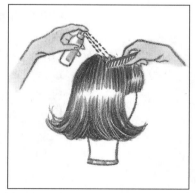

FIGURE 7–2
Apply setting lotion.

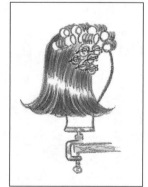

FIGURE 7–3
Set, dry, and comb out.

Buying Colored Wigs

Several wig manufacturers and beauty supply stores carry wigs of all colors and textures. Different stores have different codes for the colors of their wigs. Most stores and manufacturers use number systems to code their wigs and hairpieces. When clients are unfamiliar with these codes, they can get confused when shopping for colored wigs. The changing color-code system seems to be an international phenomenon, because from Alabama to New York the color-code system varies.

A wholesale hair store in New York, New York, uses the following system to code human-hair and synthetic wigs and hairpieces:

COLOR	CODE	COLOR	CODE
Jet Black	#1	Silver Gray (*includes silver gray with 10 percent gray*)	#56
Off Black	#1B		
Very Dark Brown	#2		
Dark Brown	#4	Jet Black (*includes 10 percent gray*)	#280
Medium Dark Brown	#6		
Chestnut Brown	#8		
Medium Light Brown	#10	White	#60
Light Golden Brown	#12	Bright Red	#130
Light Reddish Brown	#14	Gold	#144
Honey Blonde	#16	Bright Light Blonde	#613
Ash Brown	#18	Burgundy Tipped with Dark Brown	T2/33V
Ash Blonde	#22		
Golden Blonde	#24	Gold Tipped with Dark Brown	T4/144
Light Auburn	#27		
Medium Auburn	#30	Orange Tipped with Dark Brown	T2/Orange
Dark Auburn	#33		
Brownish Black (*includes 25 percent gray*)	#34	Dark Red Tipped with Dark Brown	T2/Dark Red
		Purple Tipped with Dark Red	T2/Purple
Dark Brown (*includes 20 percent gray*)	#44		
		White tipped with Off Black	T1B/60
Salt and Pepper (*includes black and gray*)	#51		

A beauty supply store based in another part of New York uses a different system to code its synthetic and human hair. Its chart follows:

COLOR	CODE	COLOR	CODE
Black	B	Mixed Gray 10 or 50 percent (*50 percent available on some wigs*)	M/G
Off Black	OB		
Darkest Brown	DB		
Medium Brown	MB	Golden Blonde	GBL
Light Brown	LB	Blondest/Brown Blend	TC
Dark Auburn	DA	White	WH
Light Auburn	LA	10 percent mixed gray in back, silver gray around the face	FG
Brown/Gray	BG		
Silver/Gray	SG		
Two Toned	TT	Multicolor (*DB, LB, LA*)	MC

A wig manufacturer in South Easton uses yet a different coding system, as follows:

CODE	COLOR	CODE	COLOR
1	Jet Black	34	75 percent Almost Black, 25 percent Gray
01B	Almost Black		
2	Darkest Brown	T4/27	Dark Brown Base with Copper
4	Dark Brown		
6	Dark Reddish Brown	T4/30	Dark Brown Base/ Mahogany
27	Light Auburn		
28	Light Auburn with Blonde	T1B/33	Almost Black with Dark Auburn
30	Medium Auburn		
33	Dark Auburn		
280	Off Black with 10 percent Gray	Brunettes consist of 1, 01B, 2, 4, 6	
44	Salt and Pepper, 50 percent Gray, 25 percent Brown, 25 percent Black	Grays consist of 34, 44, 280	
		Reds consist of 28, 30, and 33	

Some wigs and hairpieces are available in two tones. A blonde wig may have a dark scalp area, for example. Wigs and hairpieces are also available in such colors as blue, orange, pink, sky blue, purple, yellow, orange-yellow, and red. These colors are commonly used for such special events as plays and shows, costume parties, and hair shows. Some people like these colors and choose to wear them daily.

Wigs and hairpieces are available in so many colors, the client must take time to choose the correct color. The client should consider several things when changing hair color, including skin tone and lifestyle. Because some wigs and hairpieces can be too light or too dark for a client, the client should seek professional advice. In consulting with the client, the stylist or wig specialist should try various wigs and hairpieces on the client to see what looks appropriate. After the client tries a few selections, it is important for the stylist or wig specialist to explain to the client why one wig or hairpiece is better than others.

The client's lifestyle is a crucial factor when selecting hair color. If the client is conservative, a drastic color change may not be ideal. If the client is outgoing, a drastic color change may be in order. When applying color to wigs and hairpieces, the stylist or wig specialist should keep a record card on the client. This card should detail all the client's procedures and other pertinent information. Clients coloring wigs at home should write down all pertinent information. When the results of home coloring are satisfactory, the client and the stylist or wig specialist can refer to this card for continuous satisfactory results.

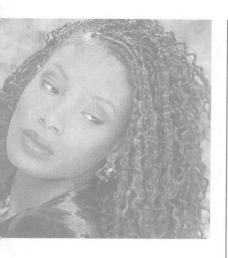

CHAPTER 8

Hairpieces

One benefit of hairpieces is that everyone can wear them. Client with all shapes and sizes of head and with any type of baldness can wear them. Some clients may be bald in the crown area only, while some may be bald in the front and crown areas. In both cases, a hairpiece can offer a degree of assurance. Hairpieces can offer a feeling of natural hair growth and a natural, lifelike appearance. When stylists or wig specialists consult with clients, they should consider the client's facial features, profile, and balding condition.

Wearing Hairpieces

Many people today wear hairpieces as part of a fashion trend or for versatility. Years ago, hairpieces were common among clients seeking help for baldness from hairpiece designers and barbers. The forerunners of today's hairpieces, called "perukes," "periwigs," and "toupees," were most common among men. Therefore, barbers were instrumental in the emergence of hairpieces. Early barbers served males only. Therefore, they were the wig-makers of early years. Today, more hair stylists are involved with hairpieces and wigs, and most salons are unisex. Therefore, most barbers are compelled to cut hair. Hairpiece wearers do not fall into any specific category; they can be housewives, actors, actresses, comedians, athletes, students, teachers—anyone. Wig manufacturers supply wigs, hairpieces, beards, mustaches, and chest hair. In most cases, there are special manufacturers to meet special needs and special demands. Actors and actresses have special needs and demands that differ from those of the average customer. Actors and actresses may have hairpieces crafted for movie scenes and for special social appearances, such as award shows and movie premieres.

Identifying Hairpiece Types

Several types of hairpieces are common, including:

- Bandeau (Figure 8–1)—This hairpiece is sewn into a headband, which is used to cover the natural hairline. The headband comes in different colors and helps hide the hairline. The hairpiece can be worn over the natural hair and is styled casually.
- Cascade (Figure 8–2)—This hairpiece varies in length from 4 to 8 inches and has an oval base. This hairpiece is worn in the upper and lower crown areas and is larger than a wiglet (see following) and smaller than a fall (see following).
- Fall (Figure 8–3)—This hairpiece usually has long pieces of hair and can vary in size. The base is usually secured in the crown area and may be styled elegantly or casually.
- Wiglet (Figure 8–4)—This hairpiece can vary in size and length and has a flat or cone-shaped base. Some wiglets have waffle

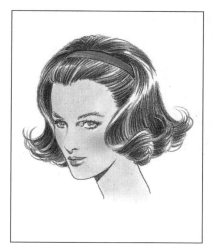

FIGURE 8–1
Bandeau.

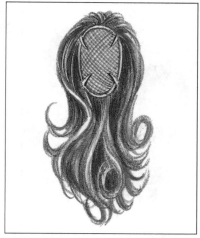

FIGURE 8–2
Cascade.

bases so that clients can pull their natural hair through the holes in the bases. The wiglet is used on special areas of the head to enhance or complement a hairstyle. It is used chiefly to blend with the client's natural hair and usually comes curly on top, full underneath.

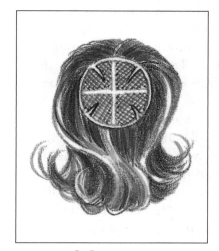

FIGURE 8–3
Short fall.

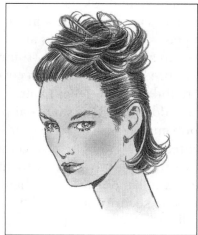

FIGURE 8–4
Wiglet.

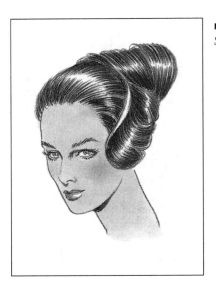

FIGURE 8–5
Switch.

- Chignons and Switches (Figure 8–5)—These are long pieces of hair that are secured at one end. They may be worked into braids or woven through the hair systematically. They are used to give the hair volume and a degree of height. They are constructed with one to three strands of hair.
- Postiche—These are small hairpieces that are usually made from angora and yak hair. They usually have round bases. These hairpieces are used widely in hair shows and hair competitions.
- Toupee—These hairpieces are used commonly among men to cover an area of baldness or thinness. These pieces do not cover the entire head, but they can cover most of it. Toupees come in short and medium-length hair.
- The "Add On"—This small hairpiece has a net base that is approximately 6″ × 5″ with four small combs to hold the hair securely. The "Add On" also comes with a small, thin band that allows the client to add hair to different areas of the head.
- The "Headband Fall"—This hairpiece is attached to a headband to ensure security and stability. The hair that is attached to the headband can be straight as well as curly. The hair can also be braided.

- The "Clip"—This hairpiece provides "instant" hair. The clip is used to secure wigs, hairpieces, or ponytails firmly. Natural hair can be pulled through the open weft of the hairpiece.
- The "Bun"—This piece is usually placed at the top of the head or in the back of the head. The hair can be braided or smoothly wrapped in a bun for a look of elegance. The bun can also come in a curly form for clients who like the curly look.
- The "Vent"—This hairpiece gives the client a look of fullness. It has built-in vents that will allow the client's natural hair to be pulled through and styled. Therefore, the client has a look of fullness over the entire head.
- The "French Twist"—This hairpiece allows the client to have a smooth "up-do" style in a matter of minutes.
- The "Bouffant"—This hairpiece has comb attachments and a wire base that give the client a degree of height and fullness. Curls are usually large to add volume to the style.
- Integration Hairpieces—These hairpieces enhance the client's natural hair. They add body and highlights to the client's style.
- The "Dome"—This hairpiece is round and small. Its hair is curled smooth and round and loose.
- The "Love Ponytail"—This hairpiece is styled and ready to be attached to the head in the ponytail style.
- The "Braided Tail"—This hairpiece is French-braided and ready for placement. It can flow loosely or it can be pinned in a style.
- The "Dread Braid"—This hairpiece is in the dreadlock style to give clients a "Rasta" look.
- The "ZeeBraid"—This hairpiece can be used to perform crochet braids on a client using a crochet needle. The braids hang individually. They are attached and secured with the crochet needle.
- Hard-Base Hairpieces—These hairpieces are made of different kinds of plastic and resin. The hair is positioned before the plastic and resin harden. The hair is rooted in a specific direction. The styling of this hairpiece is less flexible than that of other hairpieces.
- Partial Hairpieces—These hairpieces are designed to cover balding front, top, or crown areas. These hairpieces are custom-made for the client.

- The "Demi"—This half-cap wig blends with the client's hair. The "Demi" adds fullness and style to thin hair. It is usually held securely with three lock combs.

Exploring Wig History

Hairpieces and wigs date back many years. They can be seen in such movies as "Grease," which depicts the 1950s. The character known as "Frenchie" was portrayed as a beauty school dropout who changed her hairstyles with a colorful array of wigs. In the 1990s movie *Selena,* actress Jennifer Lopez wore a hairpiece many ways.

Hairpieces can be designed for all sizes and shapes of heads. They can be used for any degree or type of baldness, and their hair appears to grow naturally from clients' scalps. Hairpiece longevity is based solely on the client and the way in which the client cares for the hairpiece. A quality hairpiece can last from 2 to 5 years. A client should keep two hairpieces, in case of emergencies, and in the event one must be cleaned.

Cleaning and Styling Hairpieces

To clean and style hairpieces, do the following:

1. Ensure that the client removes the hairpiece.
2. Pour the cleaning solution into a glass container.
3. Submerge the hairpiece in the cleaning solution, ensuring that the base of the hairpiece (if present) is up.
4. Rotate the hairpiece in the cleaning solution.
5. After rotating the hairpiece, remove it from the cleaning solution and squeeze it with both hands. *Do not fold or roll the hairpiece.*
6. Place the hairpiece on the canvas or styrofoam block.
7. Using T-pins or a free hand, hold the hairpiece in place and brush it lightly. Make sure that the brush has soft, natural bristles so that it does not disturb the wig's style. Always brush the hairpiece in the direction of the style.

8. Return the hairpiece to the cleaning solution.
9. Remove the hairpiece from the cleaning solution and rinse it thoroughly. Water helps remove debris that the brush missed.
10. Towel-dry the hairpiece by squeezing it gently in a towel.
11. Place the hairpiece on the canvas or styrofoam block with the aid of T-pins.
12. Comb the hairpiece into the desired style and dry.
13. After the hairpiece is dried, place the hairpiece on the client's head and style. Use a water-based hairspray.

Restoring Color to a Faded Hairpiece

To restore color to a faded hairpiece, do the following:

1. Make sure the hairpiece is cleaned thoroughly before placing it on the canvas or styrofoam block.
2. Apply a temporary or semipermanent color. A water-based color is highly recommended.
3. Comb the color through the hairpiece, and allow it to stay on the hairpiece according to the manufacturer's directions. Take a strand test every 5 minutes to check the color process.
4. Rinse the color thoroughly and dry the hairpiece using a hand dryer. Do not disturb the hairpiece's style.
5. Make sure that the client's natural hair is clean.
6. Place the hairpiece on the client's head.
7. If the hairpiece does not match the client's natural hair, color the client's hair to match the hairpiece.

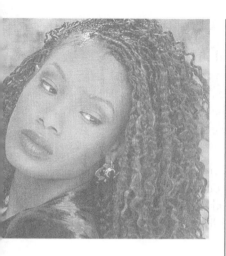

Hairpieces for Men

Custom-made hairpieces, known as toupees, are worn by men everywhere, in every region and every ethnic group. Barbers were known as the "wig-makers" as far back as the 18th century. Toupees have been popular in the 21st century, as well. Today, barbers are considered to be in the middle of toupee manufacturers and clients, but barbers are not the only professionals serving toupee clients. Cosmetologists and wig specialists also serve these clients.

Understanding Toupee Clients

Hair loss among men and women has an emotional impact. Women tend to change hairstyles for fashion reasons; men tend to wear hairpieces for emotional reasons. Few men wear hairpieces to change their hairstyles. Men wear hairpieces for several other reasons. Many of those reasons are associated with youth. Young men may seem more attractive and more successful in the corporate world.

As a person matures, the skin tends to change. Skin coloring changes. Clients should choose hairpieces in shades that complement their skin. They should avoid jet black and instead select shades in salt-and-pepper or the dark brown range. The clients' hair will look more natural and the clients will appear younger.

Baldness, whether congenital or acquired, partial or complete, can inflict psychological pain on the sufferer. *Alopecia,* a technical term for baldness, affects the hair follicle, causing complete or partial hair loss. There are many types of alopecia. Alopecia areata is a condition that causes the client's hair to fall out in small patches, leaving the remainder of the hair unaffected. Alopecia totalis is a condition that affects most of the hair covering the head. This condition is more common among males and is responsible for the loss of body hair. Many clients who suffer hair loss suffer associated pain and anxiety. Because there is no known cure for alopecia, several clients choose to wear hairpieces.

To consult properly with clients, it is important for barbers and hairstylists to recognize the types of alopecia. J. G. Bondy, author of *Men's Trichology,* outlines several types of alopecia and their diagnoses and prognoses, as follows:

- Alopecia Seborrhea (Sicca)
  Diagnosis—Primary Stage—Subjective Symptoms:
  – Tight scalp
  Objective Symptoms:
  – Severely dry scalp, accompanied by dandruff
  – Gradual hair thinning all over scalp
  Prognosis—Secondary Stage—Objective Symptoms:
  – Complete baldness

- Alopecia Prematura
  Diagnosis—Primary Stage—Subjective Symptom:
  - Tight scalp
  Objective Symptoms:
  - Gradual hair thinning over the frontal muscles on both sides
  - Prevalent in men 25 to 40 years old
  Prognosis—Secondary Stage—Subjective Symptoms:
  - Complete baldness
  Objective Symptom:
  - Complete hair loss over scalp

- Alopecia Senilis
  Diagnosis—Primary Stage—Subjective Symptom:
  - Tight scalp
  Objective Symptoms:
  - Gradual hair thinning at the vertex (crown)
  - Prevalent in men 40 to 50 years old and older
  Prognosis—Secondary Stage—Objective Symptoms:
  - Complete baldness

- Alopecia Congenital (same as Alopecia Senilis)

- Alopecia Areata
  Diagnosis—Primary Stage—Subjective Symptoms:
  - Vary depending on the cause
  Objective Symptoms:
  - Small, round thinning spots
  - Well circumscribed
  - May be parasitic
  Prognosis—Secondary Stage—Subjective Symptom:
  - Same
  Objective Symptoms:
  - Small, round bald spots
  - Well circumscribed

- Alopecia Cicatricial
  - Red inflammation near follicles and crust
  Diagnosis—Primary Stage
  - None

Prognosis—Secondary Stage
- — Same as Alopecia Areata except round spots are irregular rather than circumscribed

- Alopecia Arnata
Diagnosis—Primary Stage
  - — None
Prognosis—Secondary Stage
  - — Baldness at birth, frequently accompanied by missing finger- and toenails

- Alopecia Follicularis
  - — Inflamed follicles

- Alopecia Universalis
  - — Hair loss all over the body

- Alopecia Syphilitica
  - — Accompanies the second stage of syphilis

There are other types of alopecia, but they are rare and cannot be treated effectively by the barber or cosmetologist.

Rendering Hairpiece Services

Hairpiece clients often and regularly visit barbershops and beauty salons to maintain their natural hair. Clients must keep their natural hair blended to ensure that their hairpieces complement their hairstyles. These clients must also return to barbershops and beauty salons for regular cleaning services. As a result, the male hairpiece market can be lucrative for barbers and hairstylists.

Taking Hairpiece Tips

In 1948, Joe Carlow owned a barbershop that specialized in men's hairpieces. Carlow traveled extensively educating people on men's hairpieces, at times lecturing approximately 60,000 barbers. Carlow wrote barber books on hairpieces, hairstyling, and blow-waving. Following are men's hairpiece tips that Carlow shared.

The barber or hairstylist who renders male-hairpiece services requires the following tools and supplies:

Double-sided adhesive tape	Grease pencil
Spirit gum	Envelope
Wig cleaner	Transparent tape
Alcohol	Hair dryer
Measuring tape	Hair net
Saran Wrap or cellophane	Acetone or remover
Razor or shaper	Clippers
Scissors	Small brush
Thinning shears	T-pins
Comb	
Styling wig block (canvas or styrofoam)	

The barber or hairstylist should consult with the client before applying a hairpiece, have the client complete a record card, and understand the client's request(s). Once the client and the barber or hairstylist reach an understanding, it is time for the barber or hairstylist to give the client a preliminary haircut by doing the following. Before cutting, however, the barber or stylist should ask clients to grow their hair considerably. Long hair is easier to blend with hairpieces and gives clients a more natural look.

1. Trim the hair lightly, leaving the neckline low and side hair close to the ears.
2. After the haircut, gather all stray hair and place it in an envelope. This hair will be used for color swatches to ensure that the client's hairpiece is the proper color.

Measuring for the Hairpiece

1. Place three fingers above the client's eyebrow, directly in line with the center of the nose. The hairline should not be too low.

It should be natural looking, unless the client has a scar or a mole or another malformation that the client would like to camouflage.

2. Where the hairpiece will begin, make a dot with the grease pencil.

3. Place the measuring tape on the dot. Measure back to where the hairline begins and mark the tape measure. Be sure to measure back to where the natural hair is full. Disregard thinning hair between the forehead and the crown.

4. Measure across the top of the head, over the sideburns. The front hairline should blend with the client's natural hair.

5. If there is a noticeable difference in the width measurements, measure across the crown. Men's hairpieces are usually ordered by these measurements. The larger number usually indicates the length of the head from front to back, while the smaller number usually indicates the width of the head from sideburn to sideburn. (Always consult with companies regarding their measuring systems.)

6. Send the measurements to the manufacturing company with the hair in an envelope. Always indicate details about the client's complexion, the client's preference for hair thickness, and any other pertinent details.

Obtaining a Pattern or Model for Men's Hairpieces

Patterns or models are best when hairpieces are meant for unusual areas of the head. They are also good for the beginner barber or hairstylist who is first attempting men's hairpieces, for ensuring client satisfaction, and for building client confidence.

1. Use a grease pencil, tape strips, and Saran Wrap to measure a hairpiece. Precut the tape strips.

2. Place 2 feet of Saran Wrap over the client's head and twist the sides gently until the Saran Wrap conforms to the client's head. Ask the client to hold the Saran Wrap in place.

3. Place the tape strips across the bald area to hold the pattern.
4. Place three fingers above the client's eyebrow and make a dot where the new hairline will begin.
5. Place two dots where the front hairline will meet the client's natural hairline.
6. Place two dots in the back of the head on each side of the edge of the balding spot.
7. Place one dot at the center of the back edge of the bald spot to mark the hairpiece's length.
8. To outline the balding area and ensure the shape of the foundation of the hairpiece, connect the dots. For a strong foundation, ignore minor irregularities and thinning areas.
9. Mark the front and back of the foundation, remove the pattern from the client's head, and cut along the line.
10. To ensure accuracy and ensure that the balding area is fully covered, replace the pattern over the balding area. A foundation that is too large will not work well for the client. A foundation that is slightly too small, however, can still be used for the client's hairpiece.
11. Place a hair sample over the pattern. Use the letter *S* to indicate hair attached from the side of the head; place this hair near the front of the pattern. Use the letter *B* near the back of the pattern to indicate hair taken from the back of the client's head. The pattern is ready for the manufacturer.
12. Send the pattern to the manufacturer with special instructions as to the style of the hairpiece and any other information that is pertinent to the hairpiece and the client's requests.

Applying a Front Hairpiece

1. Clean the entire bald area with a solvent like alcohol.
2. Thoroughly dry and clean the foundation and scalp, then place tape near the front hairline in a *V* shape so that the hairpiece is held close to the scalp and appears to be part of the scalp.
3. Place additional tape at the rear of the foundation.

4. Place three fingers above the client's eyebrow and position the hairpiece above the three fingers. Center the hairpiece over the nose. When the hairpiece is in position, press it firmly and comb it into the desired style. The hairpiece is ready to be trimmed in final styling.

5. Use a razor or a shaper to shape and blend the back and sides. Also use clippers, shears, and thinning shears to blend the hairpiece with the natural hair.

6. Cut the top from front to back and check it from side to side. To avoid mistakes in cutting and blending, be sure to take only small amounts of hair off at a time.

7. Comb the front hair forward and trim it. This will ensure that if the client's hair falls forward, it will look natural. Also, when the hair is combed back, it will lay smooth.

8. If the hairpiece appears thick, use the thinning shears to thin the hair. The shorter the hair on a hairpiece, the more body the hairpiece will have and the more natural it will appear.

Removing Front Hairpieces

1. Reach under the hairpiece with the tips of the fingers and detach the tape from the scalp. Be sure the tape stays on the foundation, however.

2. Re-use the tape by reactivating it with spirit gum.

Working with Lace-Front Hairpieces

Lace-front hairpieces are intended for pompadour or parted hairstyles in which the hair is combed away from the face. Such hairpieces require a significant amount of care. The lace-front hairpiece is attached to the forehead with spirit gum, which is a sticky and fast-drying substance. After each wearing, the lace-front hairpiece must be cleaned with a soft brush dipped in acetone or some other solvent. A barber or stylist must be careful not to get acetone in the hairpiece's hair, because acetone removes color from natural hair. When the delicate lace becomes frayed, a new front must be added to the lace-front hairpiece.

Hair is tied into the lace-front hairpiece with single knots. The front of the piece is lace, but the remainder of the foundation is usually made of silk gauze. Hair is tied into the silk gauze in double or single knots. Better-quality lace-front hairpieces are made of double-silk gauze base material and with double-knotted hair.

Applying the Lace-Front Hairpiece

1. Clean the entire bald area with rubbing alcohol or soap and water.
2. Allow the area to dry thoroughly.
3. Where the tape or the lace is to be attached to the scalp, remove the hair from the scalp.
4. Attach a strip of tape to the heavy part of the foundation, near the front of the head. Never apply tape directly to the lace.
5. Place a small amount of tape to the back of the foundation to help keep the foundation in place.
6. Using the three-finger method, adjust the hairpiece to the desired position, and press the piece into place.
7. Comb to blend the remainder of the hair.
8. Trim the lace to within ½ to 1 inch of the hairline. For convenience, some clients like to wear the lace trimmed completely to the contour of the hairline. Others like the maximum security afforded by the lace margin. Clients should choose a margin only after wearing the piece for a while.
9. To keep the front hairline from lying too flat, reach into the hairpiece with the comb and twist the comb forward slightly. This will lift the hair and make it look as if it is really growing from the scalp.

Removing the Lace-Front Hairpiece

1. Detach the lace from the scalp by dampening the lace with acetone or solvent. Do not pull or stretch the lace when removing the hairpiece.
2. Apply solvent to the lace with a small brush.

3. Once the lace detaches, use the fingertips to remove the tape from the scalp. Do not pull off the hairpiece by tugging the hair. Tugging damages the hairpiece.
4. Re-use the tape by brushing spirit gum on it.

Working with Partial Hairpieces

Crown-partial hairpieces are for clients who are bald in the crown area. The hair may be full in the front and on the sides, or the hair may be thin on top and thick on the sides.

Applying the Crown-Partial Hairpiece

1. Measure the diameter of the bald area.
2. Take a swatch of hair for ordering the hairpiece.
3. To attach the hairpiece, clean the area, let it dry, and apply spirit gum.
4. Position the partial, holding it with tape and/or spirit gum. The hairpiece is ready to be shaped and blended.

Applying the "Professional Look" Partial Hairpiece

1. Make a wide part of the side, so that the tape will adhere to the scalp.
2. If the tape is previously used, reactivate the tape with spirit gum.
3. Place the partial hairpiece next to the part, and comb the piece into the "Professional Look."
4. If the hairpiece requires trimming or blending, do so using the required implements.

Applying Partial Lace-Front, Fill-In Hairpieces

Partial "fill-in" hairpieces are for clients who have little hair loss and who require little hair to make their bald areas look thicker. To look natural, front partials must be made of very fine lace. This partial is excellent for receding part lines.

1. Clean the bald area with soap and water.
2. Dry the area thoroughly.
3. Brush on spirit gum and wait until it gets tacky.
4. Place the hairpiece in the proper area.
5. Press the piece and comb it into the natural hair.

Applying and Removing Facial Hairpieces

Facial hairpieces are treated like partial fill-ins (see preceding section).

1. Brush spirit gum on the bald area and allow the gum to get tacky.
2. Press the piece and use shears or trimmers to trim it.
3. To remove the piece, sponge the bald area with a cleaner or solvent.

Working with Natural-Front, Tape-Front, or Nonlace Hairpieces

One classification of hairpieces includes soft-base hairpieces and hard-base hairpieces. The base material of soft-base hairpieces usually consists of silk gauze, nylon mesh, or plastic mesh. Better hairpiece-makers double the base material for strength and a more exact fit. Also, double-knot hair ensures that the hair remains intact. More labor is entailed in making double-knot hairpieces; therefore, their cost is higher.

One advantage of double-knot hairpieces is they are easy to clean. They may be cleaned in a mildly acidic shampoo and a water-based cleaning fluid. Pour 2 ounces of acid-balanced, mildly acidic shampoo containing amino acid protein into 16 ounces of water. This solution cleans the hairpiece and avoids damaging the hair. In addition, the solution adds life to the hairpiece and strengthens it. Single-knot hairpieces must be cleaned in an alcohol-based cleaning fluid, which can weaken the hair. When immersed in water, the single-knot hairpiece may come untied.

Plastic or nylon-mesh base hairpieces are advantageous to the barber or hairstylist because they will not shrink or wrinkle when cleaned in water-based cleaning fluids or shampoos.

Cleaning Hairpieces

Hairpieces must be kept clean, just as natural hair must be kept clean. If a hairpiece is worn, it must be cleaned.

1. Remove all tape using solvent or wig cleaner. Acetone is recommended, although any good cleaning solvent, such as a liquid dry shampoo, may be used.
2. Pour the solvent into a bowl, preferably a glass one. Place the front of the hairpiece, with material side facing up, into the solvent and allow it to soak for 3 to 5 minutes. Swish the piece back and forth.
3. With a small brush, tap the edge of the hairpiece until the adhesive has been removed. *Do not rub or scrub.*
4. If the solvent darkens, replace the cleaning solvent until all residue is removed from the hair.
5. Place a hand towel on a flat surface and place the hairpiece, material side facing upward, on the towel.
6. Again, use the brush, saturated with solvent, and gently tap the front to remove any adhesive left on the hairpiece.
7. After cleaning, the adhesive may form a powder on the lace. If this occurs, place a little water on your fingertips and, in a sliding motion, allow the lace to absorb the water.
8. Clean the entire hairpiece every 3 to 4 weeks by submerging the entire hairpiece in a vessel of solvent.
9. Soak the hairpiece for 5 to 10 minutes, then lift the hairpiece and allow the liquid to drain.
10. Place the hairpiece in a towel, and press gently to absorb all moisture.
11. When the piece is completely dry, pin it to a wig block, and gently comb it. Be careful to pull gently when combing.
12. Start from the ends and continue combing backward until any tangles that may have occurred in cleaning are eliminated.
13. Set the piece in the desired style, cover it with a hair net, and let it dry. Drying may be natural, but, for styling purposes, the blow-dryer may be used to give volume and height. The hairpiece may also be set after placement on the client's head. However, be sure the foundation and the scalp are dry and clean before placing the tape.

Caring for Hairpieces

With the proper care, a hairpiece will last for years. Clients should have two hairpieces to ensure that one will always be in good condition while the second is being reconditioned. Hairpiece manufacturers furnish instructions on the care of their hairpieces. Client should follow those instructions carefully. A new hairpiece may go through a series of adjustments to the scalp over a few weeks.

Most hairpieces are made from human hair. The hair is bought from various countries; some hair is made of synthetic fibers. The hair purchased from various countries must not be damaged. Synthetic hair is never used for lace-type hairpieces or custom-made hairpieces. Such pieces are handled like regular hairpieces except they can be shampooed with shampoo and water because the synthetics will not tangle.

Gray hairs in a hairpiece are often mixtures of black and white or brown and white. Gray hairpieces are made like other hairpieces. Hairpieces are subjected to damage by overexposure to the sun and wind. The prolonged use and improper care of the hairpiece can also pose problems for the client.

Hairpieces can be reconditioned, restyled, and recolored, if needed. Clients who choose to wear hairpieces can be assured that they will look and feel good about their choices.

Some Important Pointers on Hairpiece Care

1. Use manufacturer's tape, antiseptic, cleaner, and softeners.
2. When the hairpiece is taken off at night or for any long period, it should be placed on the appropriate block.
3. It is not too damaging to a hairpiece to lay it down without placing it on a block for an hour or so, even for a few nights.
4. It is good practice to remove the hairpiece when taking a shower or swimming.
5. Comb the hairpiece daily with a large wide-tooth comb.
6. As needed, apply a light base hairdressing cream sparingly and distribute gently. A hair conditioner and light spray may also be used.

7. Clean the hairpiece after the first week and then as needed.
8. Recommended cleaning for the hairpiece is every 3 to 4 weeks, depending on the lifestyle and activities of the client.
9. During a haircut, the client should remind the barber or stylist of the hairpiece.
10. Never fold the hairpiece. This injures or damages the hairpiece's shape.
11. Always follow manufacturer's directions for removing the hairpiece.
12. Do not shampoo the hairpiece with detergent.
13. Do not use a sharp-tooth comb or a stiff brush while cleaning the hairpiece.
14. Do not use Vaseline™ or other heavy-based hair dressings.

Selling Men's Hairpieces

1. Display different styles of men's hairpieces to show before and after versions.
2. Encourage clients to tell others.
3. Extend your services to "care and cleaning" hairpieces.
4. Be sure to have a good slogan, one that emphasizes that the hairpieces are natural looking.
5. Show photographs of different clients. Be sure to show photographs based on the age range of the client. If the client is 40, for example, show a picture of a client of approximately the same age.
6. Keep hairpieces in stock for clients to try on and to prove that their appearances can be enhanced.
7. Be sure to know what you are selling. Product knowledge is important when answering clients' questions correctly and intelligently.
8. Provide the client privacy. Be sure to conduct the consultation in private and render the service in private. This builds the client's confidence in you.
9. Keep accurate records of all procedures, measurements, and special problems.
10. Set prices accordingly. Do not take advantage of clients. Always be fair in pricing.

11. Advertise services in telephone books, on television, in newspapers, on the Internet, in radio commercials, on flyers, and on business cards.
12. Advertise different specials during the holidays.
13. Be sure to carry accessories the client may use for home maintenance.

Achieving Men's Hairstyles

Several men's hairstyles can be achieved using hairpieces (from *Artistry in Men's Hair Styling,* by the Educational Board of Milady Publishing):

The "Classic"

The "Classic" is a popular hairstyle for men with oval facial features and straight, long hair. The hair is brushed downward, with long, well-shaped sideburns. There is a wide dip across the forehead, falling casually over the eyebrow. The nape line is collar length, shaped square across the back of the neck. The whole effect is a smooth look, combed and brushed with every hair in place.

The "Curly Look"

The "Curly Look" hairstyle has the same oval features as the "Classic" hairstyle (see preceding). The curly hair is cut into short layers. Do not use the razor when attempting this look. The curls should be all over the head. A hair net can be placed over the client's head, and the client can be placed under the dryer. Brush the hair lightly, comb it, and arrange the curls where they fall easily. Spray lightly with a holding spray.

The "Oval African-American-Natural"

The "Oval African-American-Natural" is a popular hairstyle for those with slender features. The sides are styled with semisideburns, showing the tips of the ears. The hair is cut into a low oval shape in the nape area.

The "Round African-American-Natural"

The "Round African-American-Natural" has the same slender features as those in the "Oval African-American-Natural" hairstyle. The circular effect of the hairstyle is a matter of choice. The hair is cut and styled to give it the round or circular effect. The sideburns are cut to show the tips of the ears. At the temples, the front hairline is shaved into a heart shape. The nape area is round and full at about the collar line.

The "Curly Hair with Straight Look"

This hairstyle is smooth and straight, draped to one side over the forehead, with long sideburns. Hair is tapered in the nape area to fall easily at the collar line. The hairstyle emphasizes the strong features of the wearer.

The "Curly Hair with Wavy Look"

The hair in this style is waved into soft, wide waves. Sideburns are cut short to the lower tips of the ears. The nape is kept full and curly, cut to about the collar line. This is a soft look for a strong, rugged facial type.

The "Shag"

The "Shag" is popular with the young "in crowd." The hair is razor-cut for a smooth, straight look. The nape area is tapered as a thick fringe falling over the collar, or longer, if desired. Side hair should cover the ears. A thick mustache complements this style on a man. The finished hairstyle is combed and brushed from the crown to the front and down and around the head.

The "Romantic"

The "Romantic" style features thick, wavy hair arranged for a free and easy effect. It is cut to blend into the natural flow of the hair. The bangs, sideburns, and nape are full, giving a romantic effect to a masculine face.

The "Man of Distinction"

This style features a square cut, small beard, and a turned-up mustache, smoothly brushed back. A long nape covers aging necklines. Thinning hair should not be razor cut but encouraged to grow full. If the client is older, the hair may be lighter gray than the mustache and beard but can be blended with a hair rinse, if desired.

The "Athlete"

The hair appears wide in the temple area and combed off the face. The hair is brought forward and back over the ears in a wave formation. The nape is finished in a shadow-wave shaping.

The "Fashion Plate"

The "Fashion Plate" is designed to satisfy the really "aware" client. The hair is evenly cut into graduating sections that blend together, then arranged casually about the head in natural formations. This eliminates constant combing on windy days. This style is most suitable for easy-to-wave-hair or hair that has first been given a "body" permanent wave.

The "Mod Look"

This style portrays a fashionable image for the smart dresser. The hair may be easy to wave, but a body permanent wave can do wonders to obtain this effect. A left hair part goes back into a shadow-wave pattern toward a neat shag neckline. Both sides are strongly waved, the ends of the wave blending into the back just behind the ear.

The "Casual"

In this style, naturally wavy hair is finger-waved or blow-waved. A lift at the center of the forehead leads to a wave on the left side. The wave pattern continues over the ears towards the back in a free, falling, curl pattern. Full, thick sideburns turn up over the ears, achieving an easy style to maintain. The sideburns are blended nicely into the hairstyle.

The "Professional Look"

This style is best for straight hair, cut short, but full. The hair on top shows a forward movement from the left part. Scattered bangs drape the forehead casually. The thick mustache, cut even over the lip, lends expression to a serious face. The length of the nape area is optional, according to the client's preference.

The "Natural"

In the "Natural," curly hair is cut into a modified Afro style. The sideburns are full and slender, framing the face accordingly.

The "Conservative-Straight Look"

The hair is chemically straightened and restyled to be practical as well as fashionable. The back and nape areas are combed straight downward.

The "Mod Westerner"

This style is designed for the man with strong features. This style is simple, cut closely around the head into a full, wavy arrangement. The sideburns are turned up over the ears and the nape is deep, full, and wavy. The beard is shaped nice and distinct, if desired, to accentuate the style.

The "Olympic"

This style is designed for dramatic facial bone structure. The hair is brushed over a left part toward a smooth cut, back and into a straight, but long, nape line. The sides are softly arranged in waves. The sideburns are combed downward and trimmed into points, exposing strong cheekbones.

The "Traveler"

The "Traveler" is for the man who has an oblong facial shape. This style is wide at the temples with wide sideburns brushed up over the ears. The bangs are tapered to fall over the forehead in an open, scattered effect. The crown hair is shadow-shaped in the back toward the nape area. The hair should be full with uneven ends trimmed for a smooth effect. A contemporary mustache-beard, well-designed, lends distinction to the face.

The "Horseman"

This is a style for the rugged, riding, shooting, and romancing type of man. This free-falling style is brushed back off the forehead. It has no part and ends in a full nape of short turn-ups. The hair is thick, blunt cut (not razor cut) and to an even length.

The "Sophisticate"

The style is for a man of culture and refinement. The cut is conservative but with distinctive fullness. The sides are full to add width to the face. The top and crown are swirled from a right part and neatly draped about the back of the head. The sideburns are long and trimmed closely.

The "Collegian"

The hair is styled and cut to fall straight about the face. It may dip in a drape on the right side without curl or swirl about the crown and turn inward at the nape. The sideburns must not be cropped close to the skin but shaped evenly with scissors so that the shag side hair blends with the sideburns.

The "Executive"

The "Executive" style is tapered carefully and smoothly styled back from the face. The sideburns are long and close to the face to retain the style's conservative feel. The back and sides are cut close, ending in a neat nape. If the hair is a salt-and-pepper shade (gray and black), a silver rinse adds bright highlights.

The "Actor"

The hair is loosely shadow-waved (blow-brushed and combed) off the face, falling smoothly in a natural sweep across the left side of the forehead and over the ears. The sideburns are shaped to the natural growing angle of the beard line. The back is waved toward the center, as in a ducktail. The length of the nape is optional.

The "Young Trend"

This style is for the busy student participating in school activities. The right side dip is draped over the ear casually. The nape is styled toward the face and the ends are fluff-combed under with the dryer and comb. The hair-dressing conditioner is best for keeping the hair in place.

The "Pathfinder"

This style appeals to the fashion-conscious youth. The hair is shear-cut, leaving lots of bulk. There is circular movement around the crown and to the back of a right side part. The bangs fall freely and in a scattered arrangement. The soft nape line is about collar length, and the sideburns follow the natural growth of the hair, trimmed at the ear lobe.

Men who choose to wear hairpieces can wear many styles. Men who have natural hair length and just want to change their styles can also wear these styles. Over the years, the names of some styles have changed, and many remain popular. When experimenting with hairpieces, it is very wise to try different styles before settling on one. The client should be versatile and choose more than one style. By changing the hair style periodically, the client leaves others to wonder is the hair natural or not.

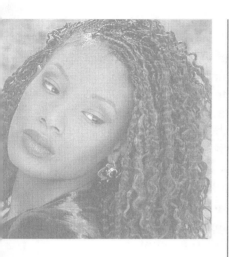

CHAPTER 10

Weaving or Wig?

A person's appearance is important, and a large part of appearance is hair. People spend hundreds and thousands of dollars each year on hair-care and hair-maintenance supplies. Healthy hair and beautifully styled hair affect people positively. Hair speaks to and defines who we are and sometimes tells how we are feeling.

Understanding Hair Loss

When men and women lose their hair, they experience grief and, sometimes, disbelief. In some ways, hair is symbolic of youth, so hair loss can make us feel older. In most cases, hair loss starts gradually and is ignored. When hair loss is noticeable, the client can be traumatized. With men, hair loss is sometimes an open topic; with women, the topic is not as common. Women may be more sensitive about discussing hair loss.

Hair loss must be discussed and often dealt with privately. Approximately 25 million women experience some type of hair loss in their lifetimes. Many factors can contribute to hair loss, including stress, immune-system disorders, illness, and heredity. When losing hair, clients should try to remain positive, not worried. It is important for the client to try to feel hopeful about the hair loss and to avoid making the situation worse by giving up and feeling self-pity.

Beginning the Process of Choosing

Before deciding on a wig, weave, or hairpiece, the client may want to try shampoos and other products that may add volume to the hair. The client may also want to try color options that may camouflage the hair loss. If the hair is shedding rapidly, use a comb with wide teeth and a brush with soft bristles. If the hair tangles when shampooed, be sure to comb all tangles, starting in the nape and starting from the ends. The stylist should consult with the client to discuss the client's lifestyle, to look at the client's overall appearance, and to check the severity of the hair loss. Once the client has had the consultation, the stylist can review options. The stylist should pay close attention to the client's personality and allow the client to experiment with different styles.

Hair breakage is a problem for hair-loss clients. The client is usually the reason for hair breakage. Clients tend to use rubberbands and ponytail holders that are too tight. This is common among females, adults and children. Parents can hurry when doing their children's hair and apply too much tension with rubberbands. The hair then starts to break. Hair loss in children can be devastating, because image is very important to children. Children can be mean to one another, and the child suffering hair loss can sometimes experience a deep depression and periods of social isolation. Children's self-esteem starts to dwindle, and they are less productive in school. Young men may start wearing caps to camouflage their hair loss. Some adults also feel less productive at work when they feel poorly about themselves due to hair loss.

Exploring Options

Today, the client has many options for addressing hair loss. Wigs can help clients regain their confidence and self-esteem and look their best. Wigs come in many styles and colors and can be styled to look like natural hair. For versatility in styling, the wig can be worn before the hair-loss or hair-thinning condition starts. The life expectancy of a wig depends on the quality of the wig and the type of hair or fiber with which the wig is made. Most wigs are good for approximately 6 to 12 months before they need replacing. It would be wise if the client purchased more than one wig, so that the wigs can be alternated during cleaning, reconditioning, and styling. Because wigs come in so many styles, colors, and textures, it is important that clients realize that wigs range from inexpensive to very expensive.

Hair weaving is a method of adding wefts of hair to a client's natural hair. The wefts of hair add length and thickness and aid in covering bald spots. The process of matching, blending, and weaving strands of hair into wefts demonstrates how the wefts are prepared. There are many styling options and advantages to hair weaving. Original hair weaving, which is painless, is the process of adding hair to natural hair by weaving the hair to the roots of this natural hair. This technique started in Cleveland, Ohio, in 1951. The hair is weaved such that no one can tell that the hair is not natural. This hair weave is easy to care for and comfortable to wear. While the hair is not detachable, the client can shampoo, shower, and swim with it.

Hair weaving can be used for the client whose hair is thinning or for the client who simply wants to change styles for a few days or a few months. Hair weaving is also used to give the natural hair a rest. For instance, when clients' hair is breaking badly and they are receiving treatments, hair weaving can be used until the breakage areas have grown back. If the client is growing chemicals like hair color, relaxers, permanent waves, and soft curls out of the natural hair, hair weaving can be used until the chemicals have grown out.

Clients with some type of hair loss or scalp problems resulting in hair loss must be careful when choosing weaving techniques. They must investigate techniques, because there are so many from which to choose. The client must also be careful not to further stress hair that is already weakened and choose a weaving technique that does not add more stress to the client's natural hair. Hair weaves can be made from various types of hair and may be bonded with bonding hair glue, sewn in with weaving needles and thread, attached to rubberbands, or woven into the hair.

Weaves made from human hair offer versatility in styling. The hair may be styled in many styles, cut in various styles, colored in various colors, and even highlighted to various levels. All this can be done without damaging or directly affecting the client's natural hair. These are the positive attributes of weaves and the features that make weaves so popular. Hair weaving allows clients to express themselves and change. Clients who choose weaves can rest assured that weaves are safe. Weave clients can swim, shampoo, shower, and even rest comfortably while sleeping, because hair weaves need not be removed.

Hair weaves must be removed and replaced based on hair-growth cycles. Stylists allow certain periods for weave wearing, but each client is different. All weave clients must visit their stylists for repair and replenishing services. These services consists of shampooing the hair, cleansing the scalp, reconditioning the natural hair and scalp, restyling the client's attached hair, and reshaping the hair, if needed. Initial hair weaving and maintenance can range from inexpensive to very expensive.

Braids and extensions are often used to help clients with hair-loss conditions and hair-fashion changes. Braiding hair into intricate patterns dates back to the days of slavery. Africans wore braids to indicate their tribes. Braiding has become popular and has demanded respect over the years. In the 1960s, African American women began to wear various hairstyles. These women experimented with Afro puffs, cornrow plaits, and the Jherri curl style. Braid styles often indicated whether a woman was married, single, divorced, or widowed. Women of diverse back-grounds, careers, and age ranges wear braids. Braids are natural and are performed on natural, virgin hair or chemically treated hair. If clients are allowing chemicals (color, relaxer, or soft curl) to grow out, they can wear braids. Clients can also wear braids while allowing haircuts to grow out.

When clients choose braided styles, they must consult with the braider. The braider should do a hair and scalp analysis on the client. The client must also realize that certain braid styles can take from 1 to 24 hours. The time depends largely on the style and the size of the braids. Mini-micro braids and micro braids are tiny and can take the longest time to complete. Several braid salons have decided to use more than one braider per client to expedite the process.

While receiving the braid service, the client should never be in pain. Clients in pain should let the braider know immediately. Pain experienced after braiding can be alleviated by misting the scalp with water or applying a warm, light oil to the scalp. These substances loosen braids that are too tight. If the pain persists, the client should remove the braids. Braids that are too tight damage the hair shaft and hair follicles.

If braids are worn for long periods, clients must shampoo as often as possible, preferably weekly or bi-weekly, or cleanse the scalp by placing the appropriate astringent on a cotton ball and applying the cotton ball to the scalp. If home maintenance is a problem for the client, the client should return to the braider or to the braid salon and have the appropriate staff cleanse the hair and scalp. Professionals know how to serve the client without disrupting the client's style.

Popular braid styles include:

- Box braids—These individual braids have square-based partings on the scalp area.
- Cornrows—These braids lie flat on the scalp. They can be long or short and can be inverted or extroverted.
- Fishtails—These braids are extended long and their ends are braided in a fishtail pattern.
- Goddess braids—These large braids are worn in avant garde styles.
- Mini-micro braids—These braids are almost invisible. They are so small that they are rarely seen from a distance. They are usually done with human hair to make natural hair look styled in different styles without the "braided look."

- Micro-braids—These small braids, usually done with human hair, offer versatility in styling. The hair can be straight, wet-n-wavy, roller set, or any other style the client desires.
- Block braids—These braids are braided in a bricklayer pattern throughout the head. They can be styled in various styles. They are usually braided all the way to the end of the hair. They are either burned on the ends or dipped in extremely hot water.

Braids can be worn for fun looks as well as looks of elegance. They can be swept up into intricate styles that can be worn to proms, formals, important balls, and any other event that is considered "after five." People of all walks of life wear braids: They can be seen on lawyers, doctors, and judges, and lately they have become a phenomenon among amateur and professional athletes. If a client decides to wear braids, be sure to investigate the different types of braids and decide which technique is best for you.

Extensions can be incorporated into braids to add volume and to increase the length of a client's hair. Extensions can be used in the braiding of adult as well as adolescent hair. Many people favor extensions because they enhance the braid styles and make the client look and feel good. Excessive tension applied to the client's hair during braiding can damage the natural hair, however. If the client has an existing condition such as hair loss or hair damage, the tension can devastate the natural hair, the scalp, and the hair root. Therefore, the braider must use extreme caution. The hair used for braids is supplied in various textures. Human hair has been favored to avoid breaking, thinning, or drying out the natural hair. Braids and extensions are removed according to the hair-growth cycle of the client's natural hair. Most braiders suggests that clients remove braids and extensions every 2 to 3 months to prevent breakage and drying of the natural hair. The braider must also consider the length of extensions to prevent clients from discomfort. Some braid and extension wearers have complained about the hairstyles being too heavy or too long.

There are various types of extensions to select from. Clients should be sure to tell the braider if the hair is uncomfortable before the braider finishes the style, because adjustments can be made before finishing the service.

Following are some extension services:

- Clip-in extensions—Lightweight and easy to attach and are made of human hair.
- Dome extensions—Blended with small amounts of the client's hair and secured close to the scalp with a tiny heat seal.
- "FibreX" extensions—Attached at the root with a nautical knot. Easy to remove.
- "Man-made Fiber" extensions—Braided into the hair. A weft fiber is wrapped around the braid to encase the fiber and the natural hair, which are fused by heat.
- "High-tech bonding" extensions—Bonding material designed specifically to be applied in a few seconds. System of extensions can be used with hair or fiber.
- Fusion—Done by using human hair that is cut off the weft. The hair is carefully removed from the weft and trimmed. A hot glue gun is used to disperse glue to the hair before applying the hair to the client's natural hair. Glue should be the same color as the natural hair and the hair extension.

Some stylists like to use the fusion method of hair extensions to add highlights to natural hair. The procedure follows:

1. Precolor the client's hair, if needed.
2. Select extension shades.
3. Beginning in the nape area, apply the "under-color."
4. Select a thin section of hair from the weft and cut the end of the hair bluntly.
5. Apply glue to the blunt ends of the selected hair.
6. Place the extension and the natural hair on a clear plastic shield to protect the natural hair, and join.
7. Comb the natural hair over the row of extensions.
8. Apply the next row of extensions, working horizontally throughout the head.
9. Comb or brush the hair gently to blend the natural hair and the hair extensions. Leave the natural hair around the perimeter of the head for blending.
10. Cut or shape the hair into style with a razor, clippers, or shears, if needed.
11. Style the hair as desired by the client.

Hair extensions create a variation of color. Extensions can offer the client color and brightness. Extensions are safe to wear for approximately 3 months. Extensions can be costly, however, especially when using different colors. This means there is more hair used than normal and a color service is rendered. Clients can shampoo their hair regularly, swim, and even return to the salon for color retouching while wearing extensions.

Dreadlocks are another hair trend popular today. Dreadlocks are believed to have originated in Jamaica with the Rastafarians, known today as the "Rastas." Today, dreadlocks are incorporated into style by means of extensions. Original dreadlocks are created when a person with over-curly hair decides to allow the chemically treated hair to return to its virgin state or when a person opts to apply no chemicals to the hair. The virgin or chemically treated hair is then twisted manually and allowed to grow out in twisted manner. Some people who wear dreadlocks believe that chemically relaxed hair is a way to enslave people. Therefore, they opt to be free of chemicals. Dreadlocks are kept clean by shampooing, and the hair is allowed to just grow. Several dreadlock wearers feel "dreads," as some call them, allow them to be free and use dreads as self-expression.

According to an article in *Shades of Beauty* magazine, entitled "Dread Heads," "when a child is born into the Yoruba culture (the peoples of West Africa and Nigeria) with a full head of hair, it is regarded as a good sign for the community. On rare occasions, a child is born with its hair matted into dreadlocks. When this occurs the child, called a dad, is said to have had his hair locked into heaven, and it is believed that he may grow up to become a priest or spiritual leader." The article also indicated that dreadlocks and hair matting can be observed in countries as diverse as Kenya, Japan, New Zealand, and India, although the traditions associated with them vary. Throughout Africa, dreadlocks hold cultural and spiritual significance, denoting tribal affiliation, religious denomination, and cultural awareness. Clearly, dreadlocks in some cultures have spiritual meaning. Dreadlocks are worn for social and spiritual reasons and to make fashion statements. Dreadlocks can be adorned with accessories to make the client's hairstyle fashionable.

The "Dread Heads" article also stated that, in Kenya, "different tribes plait or lock their hair to signify their marital status, warrior rank, or spiritual devotion. According to Hindu beliefs, dreadlocks worn by mendicant mystics, called sadhus, signified a single-minded pursuit of spiritual devotion to Shiva, the god of destruction and regeneration." In the entertainment world, we see dreadlocks worn by several artists, including Eryka Badu, Lauryn Hill, Erica Alexander, T. C. Carson, Vanessa Williams, and Cassandra Wilson. Other artists, such as Bob Marley, Karen Wheeler, Arsenio Hall, Lisa Bonet, and Lenny Kravitz have worn dreadlocks for self-expression. The following styles created by extensions give the "dread" look:

- The "Topknot updo"—Starting at the nape area, the synthetic hair is braided and the natural hair is wrapped around the synthetic hair, twisting up toward the crown. These steps are repeated on both sides and in the front. The ends of the twists at the back are sometimes crossed to give a more fashionable look, then wrapped around the front to create a bun at the crown.
- The "Fun Flip"—Using colored yarn, the stylist creates and wraps braids, finishing the ends in a pageboy flip. The result is a "Silky Locks" style (see following). The braids can then be misted with setting lotion and braided, giving the client an alternate style of a "crimped bob."
- The "Best Braid"—This style, created by braids made with colored yarn, is styled into five large twists that meet at the nape in a loose chignon.
- The "Divine Creation"—In this dreadlock style, dreadlocks are pulled up toward the center of the head and wrapped around each other. The dreadlocks give the client an elegant topknot.
- "Intertwining Silky Locks"—This dreadlock style is created by intertwining silky locks to meet at the crown, then braiding from ear to ear and wrapping the braids' ends around each other.
- "Flat Twists and Silky Locks"—Created by adding hair to natural hair and twisting the hair on the scalp toward the back of the head. A select piece of wire is used on the ends, and the hair is wrapped around the wire to give the client an array of creativity in the back and nape areas.

Different locks are created by means of extensions, and different stylists create these lock styles using various techniques. Some popular lock styles are Silky Locks, Yarn Locks, Cosmic Locks, and Nu Locks (*Shoptalk Magazine*). Silky Locks are smooth and shiny and resemble silk. They are made of braids wrapped in synthetic hair. The technique used for silky locks is derived from the Ancient African technique of "thread wrapping." The following steps achieve silky locks:

1. Part the hair in the desired shape.
2. Braid the hair all the way to the end using synthetic hair. (Many stylists take shortcuts by not braiding the hair all the way to the end. This results in unstable, short-lived locks.)
3. Using a long piece of synthetic hair, wrap the braid. (Acrylic yarn can be used instead of human or synthetic hair; it results in a natural-looking, matte finish.)
4. After reaching the bottom, seal the ends by burning.

Yarn locks are achieved in the same way as silky locks. The difference is that, much like nu locks, they are fashioned of acrylic yarn as opposed to synthetic hair. Again, extreme caution must be exercised when burning ends.

Cosmic locks are achieved through the same braiding techniques as yarn locks and silky locks. They differ in their finished appearance, which is more natural. Cosmic locks are made by wrapping the natural hair around the braided base. Many stylists choose not to braid the base all the way to the end in interest of saving time. Braiding the lock all the way to the end gives the hairstyle greater longevity.

Nu locks are essentially braids done with acrylic yarn as opposed to synthetic or human hair. The result of using acrylic yarn is a matte finish that mimics the matte finish common to locked hair. Nu locks are easily achieved by following these steps:

1. Part the hair in the described shape.
2. Using acrylic yarn, braid the lock all the way to the end.
3. At the end of the braid, use one strand of the yarn to tie a slipknot.
4. Using extreme caution, use a lighter to singe and seal the end of the braid. Acrylic is flammable and can easily begin to

burn uncontrollably. Have this done by an experienced professional only.

When wearing dreadlocks and dreadlock extensions, clients can be creative with styling the dreadlocks by making parts in different shapes. The client can use triangular bases, square bases, and diagonal partings. Client who do not desire extensions, just the dread look, can use aloe vera gel to twist the natural hair. Aloe vera gel helps twist the hair without flaking, which can make the style less attractive. The client can wear a headscarf to protect the style while sleeping. Dreadlock wearers should make sure all moisture is removed from the hair after shampooing. Otherwise, an unpleasant odor can develop.

Many clients use beeswax, petroleum-based products, and other heavy products. Super-thick products weigh the hair down. These products also attract dirt and clog pores. Stylists who provide dreadlock services should never twist the hair too much. Overtwisting makes locks thin and causes the hair to break.

Hair-transplant surgery is another option for clients experiencing hair loss. This procedure is performed by physicians and is often covered by insurance companies. Hair-transplant surgery replaces the client's hair and recreates the natural hair pattern. Some common procedures are grafting-punch grafts, mini-grafts, slit grafts, strip grafts, hair plugs, and excising, which replaces the thinning area with a piece of skin with more hair follicles.

According to American Society of Plastic Surgeons, hair loss is primarily caused by a combination of aging, a change in hormones, and a family history of baldness. Hair-replacement surgery can enhance client appearance and self-confidence. The goal of hair-replacement surgery is to find the most efficient uses for existing hair. Hair-replacement candidates must have healthy hair growth at the back and sides of the head to serve as donor areas. From donor areas, grafts and flaps are taken. Other factors, such as color, texture, and wave or curl, may also affect the cosmetic result, according to American Society of Plastic Surgeons.

Hair-replacement surgery is normally safe when performed by a qualified, experienced physician. Individuals vary greatly in their physical reactions and healing abilities, and the outcome is never completely predictable. As in any surgical procedure, infection may occur. Excessive bleeding and/or wide scars, sometimes called "stretch-back" scars caused by tension, may result from some scalp-reduction procedures. In transplant procedures, there is risk that some of the grafts will not "take." Although it is normal for the hair in plugs to fall out before establishing regrowth in its new location, sometimes the skin plug dies and the surgery must be repeated. At times, patients with plug grafts notice small bumps on the scalp that form at the transplant sites. These areas can be camouflaged with surrounding hair.

When hair loss progresses after surgery, an unnatural, "patchy" look may result, especially if the newly placed hair lies next to patches of hair that continue to thin. If this happens, additional surgery may be required, according to the American Society of Plastic Surgeons. Hair-replacement surgery is an individualized treatment. To be sure that every surgical option is available, clients should find doctors who have experience performing all types of replacement techniques— flaps and tissue expansion as well as transplants. In initial consultations, surgeons should evaluate clients' hair growth and loss, review clients' family history of hair loss, and find out if clients have had any previous hair-replacement surgeries.

Medical conditions may cause problems during or after surgery. Doctors should check for uncontrolled high blood pressure, blood-clotting problems, and the tendency to form excessive scars. Clients should be sure to tell their surgeons if they smoke or are taking any drugs or medications, especially aspirin and other drugs that affect clotting. Before surgery, clients will be given specific instructions for preparing for surgery. Surgeons will give clients guidelines on eating and drinking, smoking, and taking and avoiding certain vitamins and medications. If clients smoke, they should stop at least a week or two before surgery. Smoking inhibits blood flow to the skin and can interfere with healing.

Hair-replacement surgery is usually performed in a physician's office-based facility or in an outpatient surgery center. A hospital stay is rare. Hair transplantation involves removing small pieces of hair-bearing scalp grafts from a donor site and relocating them to bald or thinning areas. Grafts differ in size and shape. Round punch grafts usually contain about 10 to 15 hairs. The much smaller mini-graft contains two or four hairs, and the micro-graft contains about one to two hairs each. Strip grafts are long and thin and contain 30 to 40 hairs. Generally, several surgical sessions may be needed to achieve satisfactory fullness. A healing interval of several months is usually recommended between each session. It may take up to 2 years before a client sees the final result with a full transplant series. The amount of coverage a client needs is in part dependent on the color and texture of the client's hair. Coarse, gray, or light hair affords better coverage than fine, dark hair. The number of large plugs transplanted in the first session varies with each individual, but the average is 50. For mini-grafts and micro-grafts, the number can be up to 700 per session, according to the American Society of Plastic Surgeons.

Before surgery, the "donor area" will be trimmed short so that the grafts can be accessed and removed easily. A special tubelike instrument made of sharp carbon steel that punches the round graft out of the donor site is used for punch grafts. For other types of grafts, doctors use scalpels to remove small sections of hair-bearing scalp. These sections are divided into tiny pieces and transplanted into tiny holes or slits in the scalp. When grafts are taken, the doctor may periodically inject small amounts of saline solution into the scalp to maintain proper skin strength. The donor site holes may be closed with stitches. Punch grafts may require single stitches, which may close each punch site. For other types of grafts, small, straight-line scars result. The stitches are usually concealed with the surrounding hair.

To maintain healthy circulation in the scalp, grafts are placed about ⅛″ apart. In later sessions, the spaces between the plugs are filled with additional grafts. After the grafting session is complete, the scalp is cleansed and covered with gauze. A pressure bandage may be worn for a day or two. Some doctors require clients to recover bandage free.

Following are a few hair-replacement techniques provided by the American Society of Plastic Surgeons:

- Tissue expansion—Commonly used in reconstructive surgery to repair burn wounds and injuries with significant skin loss. Its application in hair-replacement surgery has yielded dramatic results: significant coverage in a relatively short time. In this technique, a balloonlike device called a tissue expander is inserted beneath hair-bearing scalp that lies next to a bald area. The device is gradually inflated with salt water over a period of weeks, causing the skin to expand and grow new skin cells.

This causes a bulge beneath the hair-bearing scalp, especially after several weeks. When the skin beneath the hair has stretched enough, usually about 2 months after the first operation, another procedure is performed to bring the expanded skin over to cover the adjacent bald area.

- Flap surgery—Performed for more than 20 years, can quickly cover large areas of baldness. This procedure is customized for each patient. The size of the flap and its placement depend largely on the patient's goals and needs. One flap can do the work of 350 or more punch grafts. A section of bald scalp is cut out, and a flap of hair-bearing skin is lifted off the surface while still attached at one end. The hair-bearing flap is brought into its new position and sewn into place while remaining "tethered" to its original blood supply. As clients heal, they notice that the scar is camouflaged, or at least obscured by relocated hair, which grows to the edge of the incision.

- Scalp reduction—Sometimes referred to as "advancement flap surgery" because sections of hair-bearing scalp are pulled forward or "advanced" to fill in a bald crown. Scalp reduction is for coverage of bald areas at the top and back of the head. This procedure is not beneficial for coverage of the frontal hairline. After the scalp is injected with a local anesthetic, a segment of bald scalp is removed. The pattern of the section of removed scalp varies widely, depending on the client's goals. If a large amount of coverage is needed, doctors commonly remove a segment of the scalp in an inverted Y-shape. Excisions may also be shaped like a *U,* a pointed oval, or some other figure. The skin surrounding the cut-out area is loosened and pulled so that the sections of hair-bearing scalp can be brought together and closed with stitches. The client will likely feel a strong tugging at this point, and occasional pain.

The American Society of Plastic Surgeons warns that after surgery, the client may feel aching, excessive tightness, or throbbing, depending on the extent and complexity of the procedure. All these symptoms can be controlled with pain medications prescribed by the physician. If bandages are used, they are removed 1 day later. Clients may gently shampoo their hair within 2 days following surgery. Any stitches are removed in a week to 10 days. The possibilities of swelling, bruising, and drainage should be discussed with the surgeon. Clients may be instructed to avoid vigorous exercise and contact sports for at least 3 weeks, because strenuous activity increases blood flow to the scalp and may cause the transplants or incisions to bleed. Some doctors also advise that sexual activity be avoided for at least 10 days after surgery. The doctor may want to see the client several times during the first month after surgery to make sure the incisions are healing properly.

According to Richard Farrell, medical hair-replacement systems are natural-looking, nonsurgical alternatives to hair loss. Farrell's salon designs and creates realistic, undetectable hair prosthetics for women, men, and children experiencing temporary or permanent hair loss due to cancer treatment and chemotherapy. The medical prosthesis can be worn 24 hours a day, while the client sleeps, showers, or swims. Clients can shampoo and style the hair as if it were natural. This hair-replacement system is said to restore the client's original hairstyle, down to the natural growth pattern, texture, and hair color. For clients undergoing chemotherapy, positive self-image after hair loss related to cancer treatment is very important.

The hair-replacement procedure conflicts with no medical procedures. Some insurance companies may cover the cost of this procedure. It is important for clients to consult before chemotherapy or radiation treatment, so that the smallest details can be duplicated in creating and designing the proper hair-replacement system. Hair-replacement salons try very hard to give clients custom fits. In Farrell's clinic, the process begins with a plaster cast that precisely duplicates the shape of the client's head. The base of the client's prosthesis is then heat-formed to the client's head shape. The medical prosthesis is created with 100 percent human hair and is custom-blended to match the client's natural hair color and hair texture. The hair feels like the client's natural hair and can be cut, combed, brushed, colored, curled, or styled in any way the client desires.

Cancer patients experience stress from hair loss and hair restoration. Hair replacement can be a major client concern. All clients are not going to desire wigs, weaves, or extensions. Some prefer other options. Some choose to wear hair-replacement systems. Hair-replacement systems and hair-integration systems increase hair density. Many clients wear hair-replacement systems while their transplants are being per-formed. If the hair in the front is thick, where the transplant is taking place, the hair-replacement system can sit behind the area of thickness and the hair types can be blended.

Hair-replacement systems often need about 1 hour of hair addition a year. Clients who are rough on their systems need an hour of hair addition every other month. Hair replacements can be performed at hair-replacement salons; some can be performed at home. Some clients choose to attach their own systems. Hair-replacement systems are most popular with male clients but are becoming increasingly popular among female clients.

Clients who wear systems have concerns that range from hair density to hair trims. If a client needs a trim, the hair system can be trimmed with the natural hair. If the hair system is on the top of the head, the hair system can be pinned away from the natural hair and the natural hair can be trimmed. It is advisable to trim the hair of the system with thinning shears. Blunt-cutting the hair of the system is not advisable. Blunt cuts with shears leave lines in the hair. Integration systems are cut just as natural hair is cut. Integration systems are less versatile, because the hairs are tied to a grid, and most of these systems require definite partings. A mesh-type system on a shaved area of the head is omnidirectional and very versatile. The client should allow approximately 4 weeks for the system to be designed.

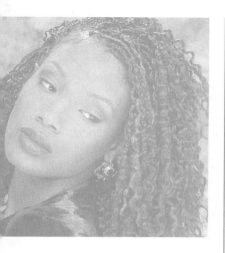

CHAPTER 11

Which Weaving Technique Is for You?

Clients who are attracted to weaving may be afraid to try it because many myths have surfaced about the weaving process. Other clients will go nowhere without their weaves. Some clients describe the weave as the "white lady of hair," because it can become addictive. Clients have made such comments as:

"I'll never put that stuff in my head."
"Weaving is the best thing to happen to the African American community."

"Weaving makes your hair grow."
"Weaving took my hair out."
"Caucasians don't believe they can wear weave."
"Weaving is too expensive."
"Weaving saved my life."
"Weaving gave me my self-esteem back."
"I can't live without my weave."

Defining Weaving

There are many misconceptions about what weave really is and of what it really consists. Weaving is a technique of attaching commercial hair to a client's natural hair to give a look of healthiness and fullness. Hair weaving is also used to cover bald spots or thin spots throughout a client's head. The client can be a member of any ethnic group with the desire to change. Weaving is discussed openly in the African American community. Weave clients do not necessarily suffer from baldness, bad hair, or some sort of hair loss.

Weaving has become very popular. In fact, hair weaving is one of the main services rendered in salons today, and the service has proven lucrative. Weave services can be costly, because some take a long time to complete. Because of the time factor, several salons only serve clients who desire weaves. If the stylist is in high demand for weaving services, the stylist cannot accommodate clients seeking such services as shampoos and sets, permanent waves, relaxers, and colors.

When trying a weave for the first time, clients must research the advantages and disadvantages of hair weaving. Clients should explore all the techniques of weaving to decide which are most suitable for their needs. Hair weaving has become the second choice after wigs to be a "life saver" when it comes to hair. Clients receive hair weaves for such special occasions as proms, weddings, formals, and plays. In the fashion world, models wear hair weaves to achieve identical hairstyles on the runways. Musicians and singers rock the night away with long hair that never changes. Models in videos dance and move with beautiful and creative styles made possible by hair weaves. Actors and actresses use hair weaves so that they can wear several different hairstyles in different scenes. The most famous talk-show host, Oprah Winfrey, experiments from time to time with hair weaves.

In today's society, hair is fun; hair is an option. Hair weaving is exciting, because with it a client can have any look. Following are some popular weaving techniques:

- Hair bonding
- Fusion
- Sewing
- Infusion
- Quick weave
- Notch weaving (interlocking)
- Netting (also referred to as a form of interlocking)
- Rubberband Technique
- Invisible tracks

These techniques may be referred to by other names in different geographical areas. The procedures themselves may vary based on location or current trends.

Hair Bonding

IMPLEMENTS NEEDED:

Hair desired by the client (*human or synthetic*)
Bonding glue
Bond remover
Variety of combs
Variety of brushes
Shampoo and styling capes
Shampoo
Conditioner

Variety of curling irons
Shears
Clippers and outliners
Thinning shears
Razor
Mousse
Oil sheen
Hairspray
Styling spray
Setting lotion
Curl wax

Pressing oil
Pressing comb
Styling gel
Blow-dryer
Towels
Hair pins
Bobby pins
Hair clips
Rollers
Roller pins

PROCEDURE:

1. Consult with the client. It is important to discuss the procedure with the client, to show the client hairstyles that can be achieved, and to allow the client to select the hairstyle. The stylist should assist the client by making sure the facial shape and profile are observed. Cost should be discussed during the consultation, because hair weaving can be expensive.

2. Conduct a hair and scalp analysis. It is important to check the client's scalp for abrasions, scratches, and open sores. Bonding glue can negatively impact these areas. Hair texture should be observed to ensure that the natural hair and the commercial hair match.

3. Shampoo, condition, and completely dry the natural hair.

4. Depending on the style the client has chosen, measure the commercial hair in the directions that it is to be applied.

5. Cut the commercial hair off the original weft, after measuring for a specific area. For example, for the client who wants to add length to the nape area only, part off side to side (horizontally) the hair at the very base of the nape area.

continues

Hair Bonding *continued*

6. Place glue on the track area of the measured piece of the commercial hair.

7. Place the hair close to the scalp. (Some stylists place the hair with the glue on the scalp area, while others place the hair with the glue close to the scalp area.)

8. Comb the hair above the newly added commercial hair over the track.

9. Make a new part and continue until the whole head is complete. (Hair placement depends solely on the style the stylist is trying to achieve.)

10. Style the client's hair.

11. On the record card, record results, special procedures, problem areas, and conditions. Also record the type of shampoos and conditioners used, color treatments, hair cuts, and any other services rendered to the natural or commercial hair. Record the time on the record card to help with scheduling other appointments.

Once clients receive bonding, they must learn how to maintain the hair at home. For the best results when applying bonding glue, make sure that the hair close to the scalp, where the commercial hair will be applied, is dry. The best and safest way to remove bonding glue is to use the bond remover formulated for the bonding glue. If doing it yourself, read the manufacturer's directions carefully, or return to your professional stylist.

Fusion

IMPLEMENTS NEEDED:

Hair desired by the client

Adhesive glue sticks

Applicator gun

Dissolving oil

Friction powder

Placement disk

Variety of combs

Variety of brushes

Shampoo and styling capes

Shampoo

Conditioner

Variety of curling irons

Shears

Thinning shears

Clippers and outliners

Blow-dryer

Setting lotion

Oil sheen

Hairspray

Mousse

Curl wax

Pressing oil

Pressing comb

Styling gel

Hair pins

Bobby pins

Rollers

Roller pins

Hair clips to secure the hair, if needed

PROCEDURE:

1. Consult with the client to ensure that the client has the proper knowledge about the procedure. Answer any questions the client may have, and allow the client to select the hairstyle. Observe profile and facial shape, and consider the client's hair color to choose the correct adhesive color for the process. Discuss cost, because hair weaving can be expensive.

2. Conduct a hair and scalp analysis to ensure that the client's hair and the commercial hair match. Observe the client's hair texture, and check the client's scalp for scratches, abrasions, and open sores.

3. Shampoo and condition the client's natural hair.

4. Leaving hair out around the perimeter of the head, start fusion according to the style, using ½ to 1 inch partings. Partings may vary based on head size and hair texture.

5. Making second partings 1 to 1½ inch above the first partings. The commercial hair will be attached to the hair within these two parallel partings. Partings may vary based on head size and hair texture.

continues

Fusion *continued*

6. Using a tail comb, make two vertical partings ½ inch apart, making the area where the hair is to be attached look like a block.

7. Place the hair designated for fusion through the hole in the placement disk. Allow the hair to hang in the natural growth direction.

8. Cutting the hair that is attached to the weft away from the weft, hold the hair cut from the weft in one hand and use the shears to cut the strands of the hair to a blunt end.

9. Place the nozzle of the heated glue gun into the hair.

10. Press the glue gun gently to push out a small bead of adhesive to the hair from the weft.

11. Place the extension under the natural hair that is projecting from the hole in the placement disk. Bring it down to meet the extension. The natural hair will stick to the adhesive-tipped commercial hair.

12. Twirl the soft adhesive back and forth between the thumb and forefinger until a cylinder is created that holds firmly to the attached hair and creates a small, neat band.

13. Once the hair is placed all over the head with the fusion, the hair can be styled as desired by the client. The hair can be cut, rolled, and thermal curled or pressed.

14. Record the time, results, special problems and conditions, and types of shampoo and conditioner on the record card. The time helps schedule appointments.

REMOVING FUSION

1. Press gently on the bottle of dissolving oil, allowing one or two drops of oil to fall directly on the adhesive connecting the natural hair to the commercial hair.

2. To remove multiple extensions from the hair, use a heated curling iron. Single extension removals are easily removed with the applicator gun.

continues

Fusion *continued*

3. Place the barrel of the curling iron or the tip of the adhesive gun over the adhesive until it melts down through the natural hair. (The bulk of the adhesive will come away from beneath the natural hair.)

   The stylist and the client should make sure that all the adhesive has been removed from the hair. If the stylist is doing the removing, the stylist is responsible for taking the time to ensure the safety of the client. If the client is doing the removing, the client should follow the manufacturer's directions closely and be sure to remove all the adhesive, because if the adhesive stays in the client's hair, other problems may develop. The stylist and the client should make no attempt to shampoo the adhesive from the hair. If the hair still feels sticky, more heat should be applied to ensure that the adhesive has melted completely. The hair may feel oily after fusion removal. If this is the case, be sure to put shampoo all over the head and through the hair before allowing water to touch the hair. This ensures that all residue exits the hair.

MAINTAINING FUSION AT HOME

1. Shampoo fusion hair extensions weekly. Select shampoo by hair type (e.g., dry, oily, color treated).
2. Use conditioners throughout the hair.
3. Do not use curling irons or a blow-dryer in the area of the extension adhesive.
4. Comb the hair from the ends toward the scalp.
5. Do not use bristle brushes. Instead use a detangling loop brush. Extreme pulling of extensions may result in natural hair loss.
6. Do not use oil on the scalp or near the adhesive.
7. If the extension becomes detached, reapply it.

Sewing in Hair

IMPLEMENTS NEEDED:

Hair desired by the
  client
Weaving needles
  (*curved, straight,
  straight with
  curved tip*)
Weaving thread
  (*should match the
  client's natural
  hair and commer-
  cial hair*)
Variety of combs
Variety of brushes

Shampoo
Conditioner
Shampoo capes
Styling capes
Variety of curling
  irons
Shears
Thinning shears
Razor
Clippers and
  outliners
Hair pins
Bobby pins

Oil sheen
Mousse
Hairspray
Styling gel
Setting lotions
Pressing oil
Pressing comb
Curl wax
Rollers
Roller pins
Hair clips

PROCEDURE:

1. Consult with the client about the method of weaving and the desired style, and let the client select a style. Analyze the client's facial shape and profile, and make suggestions for styling. Detail the "sewing method" of weaving so the client can have an adequate amount of knowledge about the procedure. Discuss cost during the consultation, because hair weaving can be expensive.

2. Conduct a hair and scalp analysis to ensure that the client's scalp is free of abrasions, open sores, and cuts. Observe the client's hair texture and compare it to the commercial hair.

3. Shampoo and dry the client's natural hair.

4. Braid the client's hair to the scalp. Braid from front to back, in a circle, in a semicircle with a side parting, or any other pattern the client desires. Some styles require the natural hair to be left out around the perimeter or just around the front hairline.

5. Before applying the hair, stitch the braids to ensure weft security. If the complete braid is not stitched, the ends of the natural hair should be stitched into the braids to ensure security.

continues

101

Sewing in Hair *continued*

6. Measure the commercial hair to fit the appropriate braid. Once the commercial hair is measured, it is ready to be applied to the natural hair that is now braided.

7. Sew or web the threaded weaving needle into the braid using stitches, as if sewing. Stylists use several stitches, including the "M" stitch, the "Fly" stitch, and the "W" stitch. If desired, use the weaving pole to help with the thread in the weaving process. Some stitches are designed specifically for pole usage.

8. Sew the commercial hair in at about 1 inch apart but not too tight. Braiding or sewing the client's natural hair too tight causes damage and hair loss.

9. Style the client's hair.

10. Record on the record card the results of the procedure, any special problems and conditions, and shampoos and conditioners, as well as the time. The time helps in scheduling appointments.

REMOVING SEWN-IN HAIR WEFTS

1. Clip the thread with shears. Angle the shears to get under the thread without touching or cutting the natural hair. Clip each stitch with extreme care.

2. Once all commercial hair is removed from the natural braided hair, use the shears to clip the stitches in the braided natural hair using the same procedure.

3. Gently loosen the braided hair.

4. Comb the natural hair using a large, wide-tooth comb to remove excess hair.

5. If the hair is tangled, start removing tangles in the nape area, from the ends toward the scalp.

6. Shampoo, condition, and style the hair.

When sewing wefts of commercial hair into natural hair, it is important to eliminate bulk. Therefore, make braids in the natural hair as thin as possible. As a result, the hair will appear smooth and natural and the client will feel more confident about the procedure.

continues

Sewing in Hair *continued*

Commercial hair sewn into natural hair can be worn for 6 to 8 weeks before the procedure must be repeated. Clients can visit the salon for regular shampoo and set services. They can also chemically treat the commercial hair while wearing it, if it is human hair. The technique itself is not damaging to natural hair, but the client's negligence and carelessness can cause damage. Also, chemicals such as color, relaxers, permanent waves, and soft curls should not be applied to natural hair on the same day wefts are removed from the hair. If clients insist on receiving chemical services, allow them to sign release forms.

Infusion

IMPLEMENTS NEEDED:

Hair desired by the client	Shears	Mousse
Bonding glue	Thinning shears	Curl wax
Bond remover	Razor	Pressing oil
Variety of combs	Clippers and outliners	Pressing comb
Variety of brushes	Blow-dryer	Styling gel
Variety of curling irons	Setting lotion	Hair pins
Shampoo capes	Towels	Bobby pins
Styling capes	Oil sheen	Hair clips
	Hairspray	Rollers
		Roller pins

PROCEDURE:

1. Consult with the client. Observe the facial shape and profile, and allow the client to choose the appropriate hairstyle. Discuss the cost of the procedure, because the procedure can be expensive.

2. Conduct a hair and scalp analysis to ensure that the client's scalp is free of open sores, abrasions, cuts, and scratches. Observe the client's hair texture to ensure that the natural hair and the commercial hair match and are appropriate.

3. Shampoo and completely dry the natural hair.

4. Section the natural hair based on the chosen style. Make partings about ½ to 1 inch apart for the area of hair attachment. Use clips to secure the hair in the designated parting area. Partings may vary based on head size and hair texture.

5. Using a tail comb, make two vertical partings 1 to 1½ inch apart, making the area where the hair is to be attached look like a block. Partings may vary based on head size and hair texture.

6. Cut the commercial hair from the weft and place it where easy to pick up when needed.

7. Pick up the commercial hair cut off the weft and cut the strands bluntly.

continues

Infusion *continued*

8. Place the bonding glue in the hair and, with the glue, attach the commercial hair to the natural hair, rolling them back and forth between two fingers.

9. Repeat the procedure throughout the head. Leave hair between rows of the infusion to cover the attachment areas. Leave hair around the perimeter of the head or around the hairline to ensure a natural-looking head of hair.

10. On the record card, record results, special problems and conditions, shampoos and conditioners, and the time. The time helps in future scheduling.

REMOVING THE INFUSION

1. Saturate the area of the attachment with bond remover. Bond remover causes commercial hair to release from natural hair.

2. Allow the client to sit with the bond remover on the area of attachment for an extended time.

3. After all extensions are removed, examine the hair to ensure that all bonding glue has been removed.

4. Comb the hair gently; apply shampoo to the hair before wetting the hair, and massage.

5. Rinse the shampoo out of the hair and shampoo again.

6. Give the client a deep conditioner and style.

Different styling implements can be used to style hair extensions. Infusion can be done on long or short hair. This procedure done on long hair looks more natural. If this procedure is done on short hair, the hair around the hairline must be left out for blending purposes.

Quick Weave

IMPLEMENTS NEEDED:

Hair desired by the client
Bonding glue
Bond remover
Variety of combs
Variety of brushes
Variety of curling irons
Shampoo capes
Styling capes
Shampoo

Conditioner
Shears
Thinning shears
Razor
Clippers and outliners
Blow-dryer
Oil sheen
Hairspray
Mousse

Curl wax
Pressing oil
Pressing combs
Styling gels
Setting lotion
Towels
Hair pins
Bobby pins
Rollers
Roller pins

PROCEDURE:

1. Consult with the client to explain the technique and to make sure that the client understands all aspects of the procedure. Observe the client's facial shape and profile. Help the client choose a suitable style. Make the client aware of the cost, because the technique can be expensive.

2. Conduct a hair and scalp analysis to check the scalp area for abrasions, open sores, cuts, and scratches. Observe the texture of hair. Compare the client's commercial hair and natural hair so that the appropriate style is selected.

3. Shampoo and condition the natural hair.

4. If desired, apply styling gel, sculpting glaze, or mousse to the hair.

5. Wrap the hair in a circular formation and thoroughly dry it, or sculpt the hair to the back with styling gel and thoroughly dry it.

6. Once the hair is dry, start to measure around the head, based on the style the client desires.

7. Place the commercial hair over the thoroughly dried hair and measure.

continues

Quick Weave *continued*

8. Bond the hair to the dry hair. (Hair is most commonly bonded in a circular motion around the head, but if the client desires a part, the hair is sculpted to reflect that style and a small portion of the client's hair must be left out. If the client desires a part, the hair is bonded horizontally.)

9. After the hair is bonded into the desired formation and the bond glue is completely dry, style the hair using various styling and cutting implements.

10. On the record card, record the results of the procedure, special problems and techniques, the types of commercial hair used, and shampoos and conditioners.

REMOVING THE QUICK WEAVE

1. Heavily saturate the client's hair with bonding remover.

2. Allow the bond remover to stay on the client's head until you feel the commercial hair loosen.

3. Once the hair loosens, gently manipulate it and allow it to stay on the hair a little longer. Gently manipulate until the commercial hair slides away from the natural hair easily.

4. Make sure all bonding glue is off the hair.

5. If bonding glue remains on the natural hair, apply more bond remover and manipulate gently.

6. After gently manipulating the hair, use an oil-based conditioner to saturate the natural hair.

7. Rinse the hair with lukewarm water to free the natural hair of styling gels, sculpting glazes, mousses, and the oil-based conditioner. No traces of bonding glue should remain in the hair.

8. Shampoo, condition, and style the natural hair.

This procedure is often referred to as the "quick weave" because it takes little time and achieves great results. In some areas it is simply called "The Technique." This procedure is often thought of as being less damaging to the hair, because the bonding glue does not touch or

continues

Quick Weave *continued*

come close to the scalp area. This procedure is not recommended for clients with scalp problems, however, because the gels, sculpting glazes, and mousses cause the scalp to itch after a certain period.

This technique is very popular; it is the most requested weaving technique in many cities. Clients who do not like to sit under conventional dryers do not usually select this technique because the natural hair must thoroughly dry so the bonding glue will adhere to it.

Notch Weaving (Interlocking)

IMPLEMENTS NEEDED:

Hair desired by the client
Weaving thread
Weaving needles *(straight, curved, straight with curved tips)*
Variety of combs
Variety of brushes
Variety of curling irons
Shampoo capes

Styling capes
Shampoo
Conditioner
Shears
Thinning shears
Razor
Clippers and outliners
Blow-dryer
Setting lotions
Towels
Oil sheen

Hairspray
Mousse
Curling wax
Pressing oil
Pressing comb
Styling gel
Hair pins
Bobby pins
Rollers
Roller pins
Hair clips

PROCEDURE:

1. Consult with the client about the method of weaving and make sure that the client understands all aspects of the method. Allow the client to select a style with your assistance. Observe the client's facial shape and profile. Discuss the cost of the procedure, because hair weaving can be expensive.

2. Conduct a hair and scalp analysis to look for abrasions, open sores, cuts, and scratches on the client's scalp. Observe the client's hair texture, and compare the natural hair and the commercial hair. Make the appropriate selection for the client.

3. Shampoo and condition the natural hair.

4. Section the hair according to the desired style.

5. Stitch the natural hair to reflect a base for the commercial hair to be attached, without braiding. When making stitches (notches), be sure to pull on the thread to ensure security, but avoid pulling too tight.

6. Attach the commercial hair to the stitched area with the weaving needle and thread. Use various stitches.

7. Style the hair with the proper implements.

continues

Notch Weaving (Interlocking) *continued*

8. On the record card, record the results of the procedure, all special conditions and problems, and the shampoo and conditioner used to achieve the style.

REMOVING THE NOTCH WEAVE (INTERLOCKING)

1. Use small scissors or shears to gently cut the thread attaching the commercial hair to the natural hair.

2. Once all the commercial hair is detached from the natural hair, use the small scissors or shears to cut the thread from the stitches (notches) made in the natural hair.

3. After removing all the thread, comb the hair gently to be sure all traces of thread are removed from the hair.

4. If there are tangles in the hair, comb the hair from the ends toward the scalp.

5. Shampoo, condition, and style the natural hair.

The client should apply no chemicals to the hair at this time. The removal of the thread from the hair could irritate the client's scalp slightly. Therefore, chemicals would irritate the scalp further.

The best type of hair for this weaving service is human hair. Human hair provides the client styling versatility. The notching or interlocking weaving system has been created to reduce bulk. If braids in natural hair are too large when sewing commercial hair onto natural hair, the commercial hair will not lie flat. This weaving system works well in giving the client a tremendous amount of body. This weaving system also works well on the client with short hair. This system is ideal for the client with short hair and a sensitive scalp. If the hair is really short, it will not be long enough to attach a braid. If the scalp is sensitive, gels, sculpting glazes, and mousses will be irritating. Bonding glue also irritates the scalp. Therefore, notch weaving or interlocking is ideal for this client. The term *interlocking* is used, because natural hair is interlocked with the weaving needle and weaving thread. The interlocking area serves as a solid foundation for the attachment of commercial hair. Notching or interlocking is excellent for clients with straight or very soft hair. These clients may feel that braids will not hold securely in their hair, and they may feel that they lack other options. The notching or interlocking system gives these clients options.

Netting

IMPLEMENTS NEEDED:

Hair desired by the client	Variety of curling irons	Setting lotion
Weaving needles *(curved, straight, straight with curved tips)*	Towels	Mousses
	Shampoo	Hairspray
	Conditioner	Oil sheen
	Shampoo capes	Hair pins
	Styling capes	Bobby pins
Weaving thread	Clippers and outliners	Rollers
Hair net used in netting procedure		Roller pins
	Shears	Styling gel
Variety of combs	Razor	Blow-dryer
Variety of brushes	Thinning shears	Hair clips

PROCEDURE:

1. Consult with the client about the weaving method and the desired style. Help the client select a style based on the client's facial shape and profile. Detail the method of weaving and discuss why the net is used in the procedure. Discuss the cost of the procedure with the client, because weaving can be expensive.

2. Perform a hair and scalp analysis to observe the scalp for abrasions, open sores, cuts, scratches, and bruises. Observe the natural hair texture and compare the natural hair to the commercial hair for selection purposes. Inform the client of any problems found on the scalp and, if the client insists on receiving the service, allow the client to sign a release statement.

3. Shampoo and condition the natural hair.

4. Use the net to cover large areas of baldness and extremely thin areas. The net usually covers the crown or top area of the head.

5. Notch, interlock, or braid the natural hair around the balding or thinning area. If the hair is notched or interlocked, the perimeter of the net can be interlocked into the hair. (The net can also be used with fusion and infusion.)

continues

Netting   *continued*

6. After the natural hair and the net have been secured by the desired method, attach the commercial hair using a combination of the weaving needle and weaving thread and fusion and infusion. For example, if the whole head is completed using the notching or interlocking technique, use fusion or infusion to add color or highlights.

7. Style the hair using the appropriate implements.

8. On the record card, record the results, special techniques and conditions, and shampoo and conditioners.

REMOVING THE NETTING HAIR WEAVE

1. Using small scissors or shears to cut the weaving thread, remove the stitches made throughout the head. The cutting of the weaving thread detaches the commercial hair from the natural hair. If fusion was used, use dissolving oil with a heated curling iron or a heated adhesive glue gun. If infusion was used, use bond remover.

2. After the commercial hair has been detached, remove the stitches from the natural hair using small scissors or shears.

3. After all traces of weaving thread (and, if applicable, adhesive or bonding glue) are removed from the head, comb the natural hair gently.

4. If there are any tangles, gently comb them from the hair from the ends toward the scalp.

5. Shampoo, condition, and style the natural hair.

This procedure works very well for clients with large areas of hair loss. The net is secured and the clients feel comfortable. Another positive aspect of this technique is that some clients' areas of baldness are very sensitive. With this technique, the area of baldness is free and not irritated. In some areas, the netting procedure is very popular, and there are stylists who prefer this technique for clients who have alopecia and other conditions that cause hair loss. The technique works very well when the client has some hair to which to secure the net.

Rubberband Weaving

IMPLEMENTS NEEDED:

Hair desired by the client
Weaving needles (*curved, straight, straight with curved tips*)
Weaving thread
Rubberbands in same color as client's natural hair
Variety of combs
Variety of brushes

Variety of curling irons
Shampoo capes
Styling capes
Shears
Thinning shears
Razor
Clippers and outliners
Setting lotion
Oil sheen
Hairspray
Mousse

Curl wax
Pressing combs
Styling gels
Towels
Hair pins
Bobby pins
Rollers
Roller pins
Hair clips
Blow-dryer
Shampoo
Conditioner

PROCEDURE:

1. Consult with the client to explain the procedure. Observe the client's facial shape and profile for style-selection purposes. Allow the client to ask questions about the procedure. Client preferences are very important when doing this technique. Discuss the cost of the service, because weaving can be expensive.

2. Conduct a hair and scalp analysis to observe the client's hair and scalp for open sores, abrasions, cuts, and scratches. Compare the client's natural hair texture to the commercial hair for appropriate styling.

3. Shampoo and condition the natural hair.

4. Divide the area in which the commercial hair is to be applied into small block (square) sections. Partings may vary based on head size and hair texture.

5. Affix rubberbands to the sections. Be careful when placing rubberbands; they serve as anchors and should not be too tight.

6. Connect with rubberbands all hair left in the section where the commercial hair will be placed. For example, if the commercial

continues

Rubberband Weaving   *continued*

hair is going to be placed in the bang, top, and crown areas, blend any ends left from the natural hair with the natural hair in the back of the head. If the hair is short, this does not apply.

7. Using the weaving needle and the weaving thread, place the commercial hair on the rubberband base in the desired style. Use proper stitches to connect the commercial hair to the rubberband foundation.

8. Once the hair is sewn onto the foundation, use the proper styling aids to blend all natural hair that is not in rubberbands into the commercial hair, if necessary.

9. Once the hair is blended, style the hair.

10. On the record card, record all results, special problems and conditions, and shampoos and conditioners.

REMOVING THE RUBBERBAND WEAVE

1. Cut the weaving thread with small scissors or shears to detach the commercial hair from the natural hair.

2. Once the commercial hair is detached, also cut the rubberbands. Be sure not to pull on or tug the hair. Cut the rubberband gently and allow it to loosen following initial cut.

3. When all rubberbands are cut, remove them from the hair manually and gently. Do not comb or pull them out.

4. After all traces of thread and rubberbands are removed from the hair, comb the natural hair very gently.

5. Shampoo, condition, and style the natural hair.

Applying chemicals after this procedure is not recommended. The rubberband weaving technique has not been around for very long, but several stylists practice the technique. This technique is not recommended for clients with very weak hair or clients with very thin hair, because the process applies a substantial amount of tension to the hair. It is imperative that the client and the stylist communicate throughout this process, as in any weaving process. The client must make the stylist

continues

Rubberband Weaving *continued*

aware of the tension level being applied to the hair and scalp. The cleaning of the client's hair and scalp is a major issue in this process. The client should use an astringent to clean the scalp as often as needed. The client should also return to the stylist for professional hair and scalp cleaning. This procedure and style can last for as long as the client desires, but the client must return for cleaning visits. If the hair starts to loosen, the client must return to the professional stylist.

Invisible Wefts (Tracks)

IMPLEMENTS NEEDED:

Hair desired by the
    client
Variety of combs
Variety of brushes
Variety of curling irons
Shampoo
Conditioner
Shampoo capes
Styling capes
Shears

Thinning shears
Razor
Clippers and
    outliners
Setting lotion
Towels
Mousse
Oil sheen
Hairspray
Curl wax

Pressing oil
Pressing combs
Blow-dryer
Rollers
Roller pins
Hair pins
Bobby pins
Hair clips

PROCEDURE:

1. Consult with the client to explain the procedure. Allow the client to ask all necessary questions about the procedure. Consider the client's facial shape and profile for hairstyle selection. Discuss the cost of the procedure, because hair-weaving services can be expensive.

2. Conduct a hair and scalp analysis of the client's hair and scalp. Observe the scalp for abrasions, open sores, cuts, and scratches. If any of these conditions exist and the service is to be rendered, recommend that the client sign a release form. Observe the client's natural hair texture to compare with the commercial hair in the style selection.

3. Shampoo and condition the natural hair.

4. According to the style selected by the client, make hair partings throughout the client's hair.

5. Place the area designated for the commercial hair away from the remaining natural hair.

6. Place the commercial hair (the invisible weft or track) on the designated area and smooth it with the fingers, applying a little pressure. Repeat throughout the head.

continues

Invisible Wefts (Tracks) *continued*

7. Once the whole head is completed, style and/or cut the hair.

8. On the record card, record the results, special problems and conditions, and shampoo and conditioners used on the natural hair.

REMOVING THE INVISIBLE WEFT (TRACK)

The removal of invisible wefts is very easy.

1. Remove the wefts with a weft-removal product. Purchase this product when purchasing the weft.

2. Follow manufacturer's directions when applying and removing wefts from natural hair.

Tips to Consider When Trying Any Hair-Weaving Procedure

1. The commercial hair purchased from some beauty-supply stores and manufacturers come sewn together on the weft, which could cause a client's hair to look thick and bulky. Split the weft to make one bundle of hair into two. Once the hair is split, the client's style will look more natural.

2. The implements listed for each procedure are important, because many stylists may only prepare their workstations for one style and one type of client. Prepare the workstation for any client in case of changes. All the implements do not have to be visible; they can be in a drawer or in a cabinet near the workstation. The pressing comb is for the client who has virgin hair and wants to try a weaving technique. The natural hair may not blend well with the commercial hair, because the hair types have different textures. If the natural hair must be left out around the perimeter for styling purposes, then the virgin hair can be pressed to blend with the commercial hair. Pressing oil and curl wax can be used in pressing and curling. Curl wax can be used to curl commercial hair, if needed. Mousse and sculpting glaze can be used on commercial hair that is already curly or wavy or hair that is straight and being styled. Setting lotion can be used if the client wants to try curly hair for a while and return to straight hair in a few days. If the client wants curly hair for a longer period, the commercial hair can be purchased curly. The shears, razor, clippers, and outliners can be used to achieve fashionable cuts once the weaving technique is complete. Not all clients choose weave for length. Some choose weave for thickness and decide to try short styles. Thinning shears reduce bulk.

3. Consult with each client to ensure client satisfaction. Ask the client questions if you do not understand the client's instructions. Converse regularly with the client to be sure that the client is comfortable, in pain, or in need of a break. Because some weaving services can take a great deal of time,

clients can tire of sitting. It is imperative that the client feels comfortable with the stylist.

4. Skin type is an important factor in selecting a hair-weaving method. Skin can be irritated by the different fibers in commercial hair. Some commercial hair is pretreated with dyes and other agents. Therefore, it is very important to ask the client about all allergies before starting the weaving service. Some clients cannot style their natural hair toward the face due to skin problems. If the natural hair cannot touch the skin, it is wise to avoid letting the commercial hair also touch the skin. The client may want to experiment with a style that is away from the face. If the skin irritation is complete, the client may not be allowed to wear commercial hair. The stylist should refer this client to a dermatologist.

5. Do not omit the hair and scalp analysis. This procedure is just as important as the consultation. The stylist must know the condition of the hair and scalp before starting any procedure. Porosity and density of natural hair is as important as natural hair textures. These factors are important when styling natural hair with commercial hair.

6. Give the weave client a home-maintenance plan. Have shampoos, conditioners, and styling aids to sell the client for home maintenance. Include combs, brushes, and even commercial hair as retail products. Make sure the client leaves with everything needed until the next visit. Factor these items into the price of the procedure. Have one price for the service, one price for the service with commercial hair, one price for the service with the home-maintenance plan and styling aids and implements, and, finally, one price for each styling aid and implement.

7. Discuss the cost of the service in detail. Some stylists choose to consult with clients at one price and perform the service later at another price. Some stylists conduct the consultation and provide the service in the same day at one price. Some stylists charge nothing for consultations. The free consultation can be considered an incentive for clients, because they give clients free looks at the salon's services. Because hair weaving

is expensive, some clients are apprehensive when trying it for the first time. Free consultations may help comfort clients. Stylists with good reputations for hair-weaving and hair-loss procedures may charge for consultations.

8. Home maintenance is a very important part of the life of a wig, weave, or toupee. Clients must understand maintenance procedures thoroughly. Clients must ask what they can and cannot do to the hair and style upon leaving the salon. Some clients spend a lot of money to achieve a look that does not last more than a few days. When this happens, many times the client and stylist did not communicate through the procedure. It would be a great achievement in the salon business if salon owners demanded that all stylists offer home-maintenance plans for their styles. Brochures can be placed in waiting areas, bathrooms, and on the workstations.

9. During the client consultation, ask the client to complete a questionnaire on general health, hair history, and general personal information. All these questions are important in building a clientele and making good first impressions. With these, clients will feel more comfortable speaking with the stylist before getting started. Some questions may be:

- What is your name and address? (Mail announcements/specials.)
- When is your birthday? (The year is not required. Call or send a card.)
- When was your last chemical service? (Know what treatments are needed.)
- Are you on any medications? (Know how chemicals will react, if they are applied.)
- Is this your first weave? If not, which weaving methods have you had? (Know if the client is familiar with weaving procedures.)
- Do you visit a salon often? (Tell if this is a transient or new client who can become a regular client or a client whose regular stylist is not available.)
- Do you use curling irons? (Learn the client's hair history.)
- Do you roll your hair? (Learn the client's hair history.)

- Are you interested in a home-maintenance plan? (Determine whether the client will return for other services.)
- Do you have any questions? (Assess likes/dislikes. Give the client the opportunity to get involved in what is about to take place and relax the client to guarantee satisfaction.)

10. The record card is very important in helping the stylist remember all the services performed on clients. If the client forgets the procedure of a particular style, a record card can be very useful, especially if the client changes styles regularly. Also, if a client returns to a salon and tells the stylist, "Do the same thing you did last time," the task is challenging without a record card.

These tips are important for any weaving technique and for every stylist in the field.

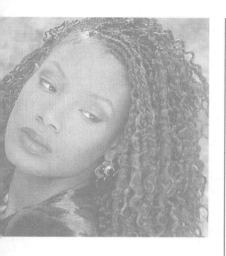

CHAPTER 12

Making Wigs

Wig making is popular in the 21st century. Everyone is looking for a better and faster way to get the best hair. Wigs have been popular for a long time. Clients with thinning hair will sometimes wear wigs on special occasions. "Custom-made" wigs, which can be constructed at home or in a beauty salon or wig shop, can be used for clients who are curious but do not want to invest much money. The wig is really designed for clients with sizing problems. Several people interviewed discussed the problems they had finding wigs that fit securely and snugly. The custom-made wig does just that and can be taken off every day or every night and put back on the head in the same style as the day before.

Wigs can be made of different colors and styled in different styles. With wigs, clients do not have to worry about stretching and shrinking. Custom-made wigs fit large heads as well as small heads. They can be constructed of human hair as well as synthetic hair. The hair can be straight, curly, wavy, braided, dreaded, or any other style. The wig constructed with human hair can be curled with a curling iron, rolled with magnetic rollers, or set on perm rods. Custom-made wigs can be styled for formal occasions or left down for casual occasions. Clients who experiment with custom-made wigs are often satisfied with the wigs' versatility in styling and security of the fit.

The "custom-made" wig is great for everyday wear, emergencies, or special occasions. These wigs are worn for various reasons. A client who is recovering from chemotherapy can try this wig. A client who is recovering from burns can consider this wig.

Wigs can be traced back to the early days of Rome and Greece and, as mentioned earlier, to the days of barbering. Wigs were popular with male clients and the aristocratic community. In early years, the wig-maker reserved custom-made wig rights. These wig makers made wigs in various colors, in various styles, and in various sizes. The queens of royal families had numerous wigs; some had wigs for every day of the week.

To make wigs, hair textures must be understood thoroughly. The most practical, manageable hair for the custom-made wig is human. The wigs with human hair are easier for clients to maintain at home. European or silky-straight textures are the most popular, as is yak hair.

Most people who experiment a great deal with hair find that the custom-made wig is ideal for their needs. With this wig, clients can have the same style every day, with little maintenance. The stocking cap or skull cap holds secure for long periods, but, if it is worn excessively, it starts to lose its elasticity. This technique is not as costly as other techniques if the client buys the material and performs the service outside a salon. In a salon, the stylist should include in the overall price

Wig-Making Process

IMPLEMENTS NEEDED:

Wig block, styrofoam head, or manne-quin head

Plastic cap

Skull or stocking cap

Hair desired by the client

Bonding glue

Bond remover

Variety of combs

Variety of brushes

Variety of curling irons

Shampoo capes

Styling Capes

Shampoo

Conditioner

Shears

Thinning shears

Razor

Clippers and outliners

Towels

Setting lotion

Blow-dryer

Styling gel

Mousse

Hairspray

Oil sheen

Pressing comb

Pressing oil

Hair pins

Bobby pins

Rollers

Roller pins

Hair clips

PROCEDURE:

1. Consult with the client. Observe the client's facial shape and profile. Discuss the client's style selection, as well as the cost.

2. Do a hair and scalp analysis to observe the scalp for open sores, abrasions, scratches, and cuts. Observe the natural hair texture for comparison with the commercial hair used to make the wig.

3. Shampoo and condition the natural hair. Style the natural hair in braids or sculpt it backward.

4. Cover the block, styrofoam head, mannequin, or client's head with a plastic cap. The plastic cap makes sure the bonding glue does not touch the scalp, if the procedure is done on the client's head.

5. Cover the plastic cap with the stocking cap or skull cap.

6. Bond the commercial hair to the skull cap or stocking cap in the style desired by the client. Bond the hair by measuring the hair for the desired style, placing bonding glue on the wefts of the commercial hair, and placing the commercial hair on the skull or stocking cap.

continues

Wig-Making Process *continued*

7. Remove the "custom-made" wig and plastic cap from the wig block, styrofoam head, mannequin, or client's head.

8. Reapply the wig to the instrument used to make it.

9. Style and/or cut the wig.

10. On a record card, record the results, special problems and conditions, and special techniques.

REMOVING THE CUSTOM-MADE WIG

1. Custom-made wig removal is very simple. Slip the wig on and off. Remove it every night before bedtime and replace it every morning.

2. Shampoo, condition, and restyle the wig.

3. Remove the commercial hair from the stocking cap of the custom-made wig by lifting the commercial hair or using bond remover.

the prices of supplies. Several wig accessories can be included in the overall price. The wig carrier is one. The carrier is perfect for transporting wigs from destination to destination. Wig luster for the shine of the wig or, in this case, oil sheen, is another accessory. Wig-holding spray can be retailed from the salon. Holding spray works fine on the custom-made wig.

The prerequisite for finding the best wig on the market is to find one that fits. The style of a wig may be great and just what the client is seeking, but if the wig does not fit, it serves no purpose. The custom-made wigs are made to fit.

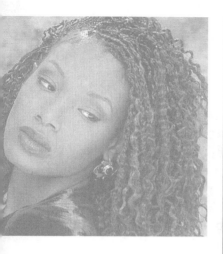

CHAPTER 13

Maintaining Your Natural Hair for Wigs and Weaves

The problem clients have with wearing wigs is natural hair maintenance. Natural hair maintenance is very important when wearing wigs and weaves. Clients can get so caught up in the convenience of wigs and weaves that they can forget about the natural hair. Some clients have worn wigs or weaves for so long that they cannot stop. These clients may feel that they do not look as good or as attractive without commercial hair.

These clients admitted that they had to wear wigs, hairpieces, extensions, or some form of locks. Some clients have admitted that they fail to get the attention they seek when they do not wear wigs or weaves.

Embracing the Commercial Hair

Commercial hair accentuates client's features and gives clients confidence. One client admitted that she would call commercial hair a "mess" and would say that she did not want or need that "mess" in her hair. This client had a nice length of hair. She could not understand why women paid for commercial hair. About 6 months later, this client's stylist asked her to try a new style. The stylist told the client that she would take the style down if she did not like it. The stylist asked the client to wear the style for 1 day and to let her know if she wanted to change the style. The stylist proceeded to give the client a weave. This happened over 5 years ago, and the client is still wearing weave today. She is rarely caught in public without the weave. She later told her stylist, "You should have made me do this years ago."

Though this client still wears the weave regularly, her stylist does her hair regularly to maintain the natural hair. Another client admitted that she was always curious about wearing braids. She stated that she started wearing her hair pressed and curled and, from there, went to a chemical relaxer. After years of relaxing her hair, and a career change, the client decided that there was too little time in her schedule to sit for hours in a beauty salon. One of the client's friends suggested that the client sample braided extensions but the client was apprehensive. After her friend made the appointment, the client got the braided extensions. She wore the first style for about 4 months and decided to try them in a different style. That was over 10 years ago, and she is still wearing the braided extensions. Her relaxer has grown out and, when she wants to give her hair a break, her stylist shampoos and conditions her hair, clips her ends, and presses and curls her hair. When wearing braids and extensions for long periods, it is wise to give the natural hair breaks between services.

Another client shared her experience with the soft-curl permanent. She had worn the soft-curl permanent for years and decided that she wanted to go back to her natural hair. She headed to the local barber and got the chemical cut out of her hair. When her natural hair started to grow back, full and healthy, she decided to twist her natural hair and not comb it ever again. Over the years, the hair continued to grow and the client had a head full of dreadlocks. This happened 7 years ago, and, today, this client is maintaining her dread style by shampooing and conditioning frequently. She admitted that she had tried dreads before going to a soft curl but got impatient and decided to try a chemical service. Later, she realized that chemical service was not for her and she went back to maintaining her natural hair. This client has experimented with coloring her dreads to be more fashionable. She tries to adorn her hair with such accessories as scarves, beads, and decorative hair pins. This client feels that her hair is the healthiest it has ever been. She feels a sense of "freedom," she said. She also said she is "free from chemicals, free from the curling iron, and free from pressing combs and thermal curlers."

Clients with virgin hair can wear dreads, presses and curls, and wigs and weaves. If a client wears a thermal press and curl and wants to change her style or just give her hair a rest from the thermal irons, the client can receive any one of the weave services mentioned in preceding chapters. The client can wear a commercial wig or a custom-made wig. The client can try a weave or extensions. While deciding, the client can maintain her thermal press and curl service between visits to break up the routine and give her hair the breaks it needs.

Clients with relaxers can use wigs and weaves as an option. Over a period of time, relaxers can be deadly to the hair. The hair loses its elasticity and life. The hair needs cutting, but many clients forbid stylists from cutting their hair. After a while of not cutting the hair and constantly retouching the new growth with relaxer, the hair starts to break and shed. At this time, the hair needs a break from the chemical. Some clients opt for hair cuts, while others receive some type of weaving service. Some clients go as far as receiving a hair cut and a weaving service or wear a wig. If the hair is relaxed and the client is going to wear a wig or a weave, the client needs to be sure to shampoo and condition with the proper supplies. The client with the chemical service really needs a professional stylist to treat chemically treated natural hair. Clients doing hair at home can damage the hair further, because clients do not always understand the chemical makeup of their hair or the products they are using. There-fore, if clients use products that can dry or damage the hair, wig and weaves are going to be coverups for damaged natural hair. If natural hair is damaged and ignored by the client, it will come out. Once the natural hair starts to fall out, a wig or a weave is not an option. It is mandatory. If a client is going to allow relaxer to grow out of the hair, wig and weaves are great options. The hair can look good while the chemical service is growing out. Clients who choose braids must be sure to communicate with the braider, because excess tension on relaxed hair can result in hair loss. Also, negligence of natural hair can result in hair loss. If a client with a permanent wave or naturally curly hair decides she wants a straight look, she can try a weave service or a straight styled wig. In the movie "Eye of the Beholder," Ashley Judd changes her look with different straight wigs. Wigs are available in many straight styles, long and short. The client who has a permanent wave or natural curly hair can wake up any morning and say, "I'm going straight today."

The client who has color in the natural hair may decide to try another color. It may be too soon to apply another color to the natural hair, however. If so, the client may want to try a wig or a weave. If the client does decide to try a wig or a weave, the client must understand that color-treated hair needs a lot of nourishment. The hair needs routine shampooing and conditioning treatments to stay healthy. Negligence will result in hair loss. Color-treated hair on clients who have combinations of chemical services can be problematic. Chemical combinations can consist of relaxer and color, permanent wave and color, soft curls and color, and texturizers and color. If these combinations are in a client's natural hair, the client must be sure that the hair is being treated properly. Clients should not try to treat these natural-hair combinations at home. They should visit a professional stylist who can educate the clients about home maintenance.

If the client wants to change colors, the wig could be purchased in the color desired or the weave style could be performed in the color desired by the client. The client could take these options into consider-ation and once decided, could allow the natural hair to grow out of the existing color and back to the natural color. At this time, wigs and weaves can be deleted from the hair equation and the client can color the natural hair as desired. If the client is a first-time color client, the client may seem apprehensive about trying the color. If this is the situation, the stylist or wig specialist may want to suggest a wig or weave service. The client can then try the new color before coloring the natural hair. After the client wears the new color, the client may decide that the new color is not for her, and her natural hair is saved from the chemical that may have had to be applied and reapplied to the client's hair in the hope of achieving the correct color. Not only are wigs and weaves fashionable, they are helpful in saving the natural hair.

Maintaining the Natural Hair

Maintaining the client's natural hair is very important and should be the primary goal in the beauty business. Anyone who desires long or short, thick hair can have it. Any client who wants curly, straight, wavy, colored, locked, or spiked hair can have it in a matter of a few hours. Hair care is starting to get back to the basics. If the client has natural hair, the stylist should make every effort to make sure that the hair remains healthy. Therefore, a wig, a weave, or extensions remain options. Many people are losing their hair, including some who are going to stylists regularly. This should not be happening. Stylists are going to take a little more time to educate themselves on hair maintenance and to help educate clients.

"Shop hopping" can threaten client's natural hair because all stylists do not use the same products. Some products are not formulated to be used with other products. The clients in most cases are not familiar with all the products on the market. Therefore, they cannot tell the next stylist what the previous stylist used. When this happens, the natural hair is subjected to damage. If there is going to be a stylist change, the change should be within the same salon. The staff in the salon should be a team. The salon owner would be pleased to know that the business has not left the establishment.

Another advantage for making an internal salon change is that the client is already used to visiting this particular salon. Clients will also feel comfortable knowing that if the regular stylist is busy, in case of emergency, there is someone in the same establishment who can serve them. Yet another advantage of staying in the same salon is that everyone in the salon is possibly using the same products. If the products used on the client's natural hair are working for the client, it will be reassuring for the client to know that the treatment of her natural hair will be consistent.

Some clients have worn different styles all of their lives and decide to start over and cut their hair really short, almost bald. In the last decade, many clients have done this, for whatever reason. Some clients say that cutting the hair off and starting over is a spiritual change. Some clients cut their hair for a fashion change; others cut their hair because it is damaged. Some cut their hair because they want to "start over" or "have another fresh start" in regards to hair maintenance. Such clients tax their hair. Natural hair can only take so much. It needs rest and nourishment, just as the body does. Diet is important in maintaining healthy, natural hair. Lifestyle is also important in maintaining natural hair. Such elements as exercise, proper rest and relaxation, lack of stress, and nutrition are all important in maintaining natural hair.

Wearing different wigs and weaves is great and can help preserve natural hair, but overindulgence in hairstyles, including pulling the natural hair too tight, applying an excessive amount of bonding glue to the hair shaft, removing bonding glue or weaving thread improperly, and removing the fusion and infusion improperly, can all result in hair loss. Wearing wigs for excessively long periods and failing to shampoo and condition the natural hair can result in hair loss. Wearing braids too tight and too long without shampooing and conditioning can also result in hair loss.

Recently, a parent's negligence in attending to a child's hair that had been braided for a long period resulted in death. The child, a fifth grade student, wanted the new braid style that was popular with her peers. The child's mother, who was a single, working parent, decided to allow the child the new hairstyle. The child wore the braids for approximately 5 months with little or no attention from the mother. The mother neglected to keep the child's hair conditioned and shampooed. After a few months, the child started to complain of constant headaches. Her mother ignored the complaints as attention seeking. After a few more weeks, the child again complained about the headaches, but the mother again ignored the complaints. The child then went to a teacher at her school and complained about the excruciating pain in her head. Before the teacher could address the complaint, the child fell to the floor and died. She died due to hair negligence. A spider had gotten to the base of the child's braids, started to eat away at the child's scalp, and hatched other spiders in the fifth grader's head.

Braiding itself is not bad. Neglect of commercial or natural hair, for any time at all, will cause some type of problem, however. All clients must maintain their natural hair and their commercial hair. Through hair maintenance, we show who we are. Physical appearance is part of the first impression. Maintain your natural hair and make good first impressions, at all times.

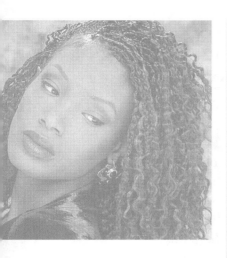

CHAPTER 14

Specialty Salons

Specialty salons are very popular today. General salons not operating as full-service salons are starting to cut overhead and focus just on the services they specialize in, not everything. Some stylists open specialty salons because they really enjoy performing particular skills.

Identifying the Keys to Success

Just as in any other salon, some basic elements make the specialty salon a success. These elements are common among professional salons. The first relates to client dislikes.

Avoiding Client Dislikes

Stylists Who Are Not Creative Enough. Some clients feel that stylists are not innovative and take no initiative when creating client styles. Clients leave unsatisfied because they wanted something different but did not know how to express it to the stylist.

Long Wait Time. The most common complaint clients have about salons is a long wait time. This seems to be a problem nationwide. Stylists should make appointments according to the service. A stylist should not make appointments for a lot of weaving services in one day, for example. While performing a weave, the stylist can encounter several problems, such as knotting of the thread and glue clogging.

Tipping. Clients sometimes feel that prices are too high and do not tip the stylist as a result. Some clients are offended when stylists ask for tips. Tipping is customary and appreciated.

Stylist Appearance. Several myths are related to hairstylist appearance. One is, "Hairstylists never comb their hair." Although this is a myth, it is common. Some hairstylists do not represent the industry to the best of their abilities. Clients watch and, in many cases, look to the hairstylist for trends. Therefore, hairstylists should keep their personal appearances immaculate. Hairstylist appearance should mirror hairstyle service. It may help the stylist or wig specialist's clientele to see the hairstylist or wig specialist wearing a wig or a weave.

Gossip. Gossip is one of the main reasons businesses fail. In a specialty salon serving clients wearing wigs and weaves, it is important for clients to be comfortable. Clients with some sort of hair loss expect stylists and wig specialists to be compassionate as well as private. Clients may not be ashamed of their conditions, but they can be sensitive about them. Clients do not expect stylists to tell everyone in the salon about the clients' conditions. It is unprofessional for stylists to discuss clients with other clients. One stylist who gossips can ruin a whole salon. Clients seek salons that eliminate gossiping hairstylists.

Advance Appointments. Some clients feel that their appointments are made too far in advance. These clients feel that stylists should not make appointments 3 to 4 months in advance, but clients do not always understand how busy some stylists are in specialty salons. Because of the services they render, specialty salons have large numbers of clients with standing appointments. Weave and wig clients are very faithful when they find stylists or wig specialists who can service them and are sensitive to their needs. Therefore, making appointments in specialty salons can take some time.

Overall Salon Appearance. Salon owners are not always as focused on the appearance of the salons as they are on the appearance of clients. Some salon owners feel that as long as the inside of the salon has all the equipment necessary for the stylists to work, their job is done. Appearance starts on the outside of the establishment. When clients drive to the salon, they observe their surroundings. They usually start with the outside, including advertisements, paint or types of bricks, siding, window displays, and the parking lot or parking area. When clients enter the door, they evaluate the inside of the establishment. Therefore, the salon should always remain clean. The salon should have a receptionist who represents the establishment. The receptionist is the first person the client sees. The specialty salon should also have photographs and advertisement of the services in which the salon specializes. If the salon has a great appearance overall, clients tell everyone they know, which gives the salon a great reputation. Once the salon has a great reputation, the salon has great business.

Client Protection. Some stated, "Stylists don't care about clients." Most clients interviewed felt the stylists today are always in a hurry and do not protect the clients the way they should. One client mentioned, "Every time I visit the salon, my clothes get wet." The client went on to express that if the stylist cared about her, this would not happen every time. Another client mentioned, "The stylist showed no concern about wetting my clothes, no apology, nothing. The sad part about this is, I like her work." Clients watch everything stylists do and start to trust the stylists or wig specialists after several visits. Stylists and wig specialists should make clients their first priority. When performing a wig or weave service, the stylist must protect the client by making sure all the hair wefts (tracks) are covered, by making sure the weave or braids are not too tight or uncomfortable, and, if the client is wearing a wig, making sure the wig fits properly.

Jealousy among Salon Staff. Relationships among salon staff can often impact clients. If clients notice animosity among staff, it can cause discomfort among clients. Clients stated that they had left salons for this reason, even though they like their stylist's work. Clients felt they were under too much pressure to enjoy their salon visits. Clients visit salons to alleviate stress, not to be subjected to stress.

Pushy Retailing. Clients are often offended when stylists seem to push products on them that they do not need. Clients interviewed said they can always tell when a stylist is sincere and when a stylist is trying to meet a quota. Clients are very perceptive. In specialty salons, it is imperative to have retail items visible. The items should be items the stylist knows the clients need for home maintenance. Clients who are educated while receiving the wig or weave service, or any other hair service, will ask the stylist about retail items. When this happens, the stylist does not have to make a sell.

Despite these complaints, clients like a lot of things about salons. When clients offer constructive criticism of salons, it can help the salon. The constructive criticism can help because clients often observe things about salons that are not observed by the salon owner and staff. Once the constructive criticism is accepted and evaluated, the salon owner and staff can start to make a change. Positive changes lead to positive results.

Many salons are doing what they need to do to be successful. Clients love to visit these salons because of the salons' positive attributes. They feel like going to their favorite salons is truly rewarding. These clients feel the salons are areas to visit for emotional retreats and renewals. Some clients stated that visiting their salons was a "spiritual revival for their souls," "an experience I'll never forget," "a time to really, really relieve stress," "a second home," "truly magical," "a place of privacy," and "the best place on earth." These satisfied clients expressed the attributes they liked about their salons.

Providing Client Likes

Good Waiting Area. The waiting area, which gives the vibe of the entire salon, should be relaxing. The décor of the waiting area should not be gaudy or too colorful. Music, if played, should be relaxing. Salon books should be nice, not torn. An appropriate amount of sitting space should be available. The waiting area can be an area in which to educate the clients by playing educational videos. For example, if a salon specializes in wigs and weaves, the videos should be about wigs and weaves, including before and after pictures, a home-maintenance plan, and different wig and weave options.

A Cheerful Staff. Clients feel good if stylists seem to feel good. Stylist attitude regulates the mood of the salon. Salon staff should try their best to display cheerfulness. If the staff have bad attitudes, they usually attract clients with bad attitudes. When staff are cheerful, they can make clients feel better. The staff or stylist can make clients change their outlooks without even realizing it. Some clients visit their stylists to seek answers about personal problems and other situations. Being cheerful makes the client feel that the stylist is approachable and that the client can relax.

Well-Skilled Staff. Clients like nothing more than well-trained staff. Clients feel a sense of dignity and pride when visiting a salon like this. The staff carries "a certain air about them," said one client. Another client who is very pleased with her salon said she was "just honored to be a part of her salon's family." Clients all over share the feeling that salons with staffs "can carry their own." Some stylists, who are not part of this setting, want to be part of it. It is very reassuring to salon owners and to clients when stylists are educated and properly trained. Clients have no problem paying for services, buying retail items, or tipping when stylists or wig specialists "know what they know."

Client Sacrifices. Today, clients are as busy as ever juggling family and career. These clients often need sympathetic stylists. This does not mean that stylists should feel sympathy for the client so that the client takes advantage of the situation, but many clients have times when emergencies occur and they need the stylist or wig specialist to make an exception regarding appointment time. Many stylists understand because they are also juggling families and careers. When stylists or wig specialists make sacrifices for their clients, the clients are often most appreciative, and the stylists or wig specialists will be on the road to client longevity. Stylists or wig specialists who plan to remain in the industry must realize that sacrifices are the key to major success.

Client Satisfaction. Clients expressed the importance of being satisfied when leaving a salon. Many stylists and wig specialists do not communicate well with their clients, and problems occur. Many other stylists and wig specialists pay close attention to their clients. Paying close attention means listening to what clients say. Clients sometimes confuse a stylist or wig specialist, because they do not use the correct terminology. The stylist or wig specialist must then play the "guessing game." The stylist or wig specialist should never play the "guessing game," however, especially when it involves hair cutting. Most clients know exactly what they want when they walk in the door. Some, however, have no idea. The stylist or wig specialist must know the client to offer the client satisfaction.

Paying Attention to Details. One of the most positive attributes clients expressed was the fact that their stylist or wig specialist pays close attention to the small things. "If there is a hair out of place, the stylist will see it," said one client. "My stylist always cleans dried residue from setting lotions and sculpting gels left on my skin," explained another. "If the shampoo tech in training didn't rinse me well, my stylist will do it herself," said another client. A regular weave wearer stated, "My stylist always insists on purchasing the best hair for my styles." The little things a stylist or wig specialist does can have a major impact on building client relations as well as building a clientele.

Professional Image. Clients have expressed their feelings about dress codes. Many like the opportunity to differentiate the stylist or wig specialist from the clients. In some salons, clients and staff dress in the same attire. A client who visited a salon for the first time had a hard time identifying who was employed and who was not. Many salons that do not have dress codes have said that they run fine. Some salons that did not have dress codes adopted them later and reported a boost in clientele. The salons' clients expressed feelings of being pleased with the change.

Good Lighting. Many clients like the lights displayed in salons. The lights are much brighter than their lights at home. The clients are allowed to see their true hair color or wig or weave color. Hair texture and hair and scalp abrasions can be observed closely in a well-lit salon. Some clients expressed that they like a combination of lights. They liked soft, relaxing lights in the waiting area, the shampoo area, and the dryer areas, because these areas are the areas where they spend most of their time. Some clients expressed that they liked soft lights in the bathroom, while others expressed that they liked bright lights so they could evaluate their hairstyles or wig styles after the stylist or wig specialist finished. It is obvious that lighting is important in any salon, but client input can be very helpful.

Clean Smells. Clients expressed the joy of smelling freshness when visiting a salon. Often, salons smell like chemicals, which is not so pleasant. Clients do not like entering salons that smell bad. If the clients are stressed when they enter the salon, foul odors do not help. In performing some weaving services, such as fusion, there is a very mild odor from the adhesive. In performing chemical services, such as permanent waving, there is somewhat of a foul odor. In situations like these, there should be an abundant amount of ventilation in salons and a designated area for services.

Updated Magazines and Books. Salons that subscribe to the latest magazines and buy the latest books are popular among clients. Clients depend on these salons to offer the latest trendy styles. A nice variety of magazines and books can also help entertain clients. Often, magazines are entertainment tools for children and young adults as well as older clients. One client said, "My stylist has coloring books for children in her salon and it really helps entertain my children." She added, "Visiting the salon has become a family affair." One client shared, "My preteen daughter really enjoys looking through the bridal magazines that my stylist carries in her salon." Another client expressed, "I just love reading the self-help books my stylist has made available, because, otherwise, I wouldn't have time to read them." Most salon owners and staff members do not understand the role magazines and books play in building salon credibility. These materials can play an integral role in increasing salon business.

Kept Appointments. Dependable and reliable stylists and wig specialists rarely have problems building clientele. Clients expressed gratitude to stylists and wig specialists with reputations for keeping appointments and minimizing cancellations. Some clients said, "I know my stylist like clockwork. She is always on time." Another satisfied client said, "If I miss my appointment, I pay anyway." "I pay because I want to keep my standing appointment and I love my stylist." A wig client said,

"My stylist always keeps my appointment and is always introducing me to new wig styles."

Therefore, keeping appointments is an important attribute for any stylist or wig specialist. One stylist said, "Because I am dependable and keep appointments, my clients sent me on a cruise as a gesture of appreciation."

Staying Ahead of Clients

The salon owner and staff must investigate ways to stay ahead of public attitude. Salon business depends on the public. Some stylists argue that they are not public servants. Others disagree. Whether stylists want to believe this concept or argue it, the most important aspect to surviving in the beauty and barbering industry is "staying ahead of the clients." Some tips for staying ahead of clients follow.

Ask Other People. Stylists and wig specialists should ask other people for input and feedback about the services they perform. Whether the information is good or bad, it should be taken in by the stylist or wig specialist and processed. If the information is bad, it allows the stylist or wig specialist to listen for future information of this sort. If more information is received, the stylists or wig specialists can start to reevaluate themselves and their businesses. If the information is good, the stylists or wig specialists should focus on making their business better.

Always Listen to Constructive Criticism. One of the best ways to improve your business is to process constructive criticism continuously. It is an opportunity to turn negative into positive. Although clients are not always right, they can still be helpful. They can help the stylist or wig specialist look at situations differently. Stylists or wig specialists must realize that they can always improve. Even the "best salons" can always improve on something.

Watch the Competitor. Even the salons that seem to be doing everything right still need to keep an eye on the competition. Good competition is not a "bad thing." Stylists from different salons should interact and share ideas about what is working in their businesses and what is not. Salon owners should also interact and share business tactics. Competition is good as long as it remains positive and everyone involved benefits from it.

Read All Professional Publications. By reading professional publications, wig and weave specialists, as well as hairstylists, can keep up with the latest trends. Professional publications detail hair shows in different areas, as well as educational classes. To stay ahead of the clients, stylists and wig and weave specialists must learn new techniques and experiment on new clients. Clients look forward to stylists and wig specialists going to new educational events, because they feel the stylists or wig specialists will have more to offer upon returning. Reading professional publications also allows stylists or wig specialists to visualize what other professionals in the industry are doing to make their businesses successes.

Rewarding Salon Staff Members. Salon owners should notice if a stylist or wig specialist is doing exceptionally well. Salon owners should reward the staff members who take initiative for the salon. The staff member who has an overflowing clientele should also be rewarded. By rewarding hardworking staff members, the salon will grow. The staff member who is not producing fully will want to produce. This practice leads to growth in clientele for the salon and makes "happy" salon owners.

Salon Meetings. Some salon owners fail to communicate with their staff. Salon owners need to take time to meet with salon staff. Staff members can often see things and hear comments the salon owner will generally miss. In salon meetings, updated information can be shared, product knowledge can be taught, problems can be solved, and success stories can be told. In having salon meetings, the shop can stay ahead of the clients and the competitors. For example, if a wig specialty salon conducts a meeting, the latest wigs on the market can be introduced. In a weave specialty salon, the latest weaving technique can be taught to the staff. Open communication between salon staff members is very helpful in keeping up with the trends and staying ahead of clients.

Owning and Operating a Salon

Owning and operating a salon is the ultimate goal for many aspiring cosmetology and barbering students, as well as many nail technology and esthetics students. If owning and operating a salon is what an individual is aspiring to do, it is important that the individual understands what is entailed. There are numerous responsibilities involved with ownership. Not everyone is conditioned to tolerate all the demands placed on the individual. Owning and operating a salon can be a very rewarding experience. There are very positive aspects of ownership. Several salon owners interviewed expressed warm feelings about ownership. One owner said, "In ownership, make sure the good always outweighs the bad, and a person will be fine." In owning a specialty salon and any other salon, the name of the game is "staying ahead of the clients."

Planning a Budget for a Specialty Salon

Opening a specialty salon and a general salon involves a tremendous amount of responsibility. The owners of these salons should have budget plans before embarking on this task. Many salon owners do not properly plan their moves. Therefore, they do not have the success that they expect. A budget is very helpful in planning. A budget allows owners to know what they can and cannot afford. Many salon owners go into owning and operating with "blinders on" and underbudget for the expenses ahead.

Some of the largest salons do not offer the services the actual building allows them to offer, because they are inadequately equipped. The owner and operator of the salon may have failed to plan and establish a budget. This is also obvious in the smallest salons. Many large buildings have the space to offer more services, but the staff does not have the proper equipment. These situations can cause problems among staff. The morale of the staff employed in the salon is very low. They may feel dismay, because they have the skills to perform services but no space or equipment. Many salon staffs suffer from these feelings, especially in booth-rental settings. When stylist or wig specialists pay booth rent, they often rent space and, in some salons, they can use the whole facility.

Public relations is an element of success that is often left off the budget list. Public relations is very important to the success of any business. The budget for public relations should be established by asking the following questions:

- What are the needs of the salon?

- What are some elements/items that are appealing to the clients?
- Who is my competition?
- How far is my closest competitor?
- What services will I offer in my business?
- Will I use booth rental, commission, or salary?
- What is the most effective media for my business?
- How much will I invest in advertising?
- Who will be our clients?
- What are the long-term needs of this salon?
- Have I analyzed the target area enough?
- How much money should I set aside for emergencies?
- Is there adequate parking?
- Is the salon located where it is easy to access?
- What type of organizational staff will I employ?
- Will I work in the salon or play the role of owner/overseer?

All these questions, and more, should be asked when preparing a budget. The budget in some salons includes payroll. If a salon owner does not take these issues into consideration before opening a salon, the salon is doomed. Once the salon business fails, it is very hard to regroup. Clients will start to communicate with other clients about competing businesses. If the clients realize your business is failing and know the reasons the business is failing, the entire community will know, especially if it is a small community. In large cities, salon owners and operators make changes more often than stylists in small areas. When planning to open a specialty salon or a general salon, always prepare a budget.

Advertising the Specialty Salon

Good advertising is a great way to bring business to the salon. Radio, television, billboards, business cards, flyers, and word of mouth are popular ways to advertise. It is often said, "The best way to advertise your business is by word of mouth." Many people believe, "Seeing is believing." If potential clients can see and feel your work, they are impressed and will follow through by asking, "Who did your style?," "Where is the person located?," "Do you have a phone number?," "Can you give me directions?" These are the questions generally asked by potential clients when they see the work of a stylist or wig specialist on a client.

Radio and television can really help your business become a success. The radio reaches listeners of all ages, as well as those who do not watch television. People who watch abundant television and do not listen to the radio can see your advertisement through commercials. Salon owners should "showcase" their salons on television. Clients will be allowed to see others receiving the services they may want. If the salons are nicely decorated, the television viewer will be allowed to see the atmosphere of the salon. The radio station chosen for the advertisement of the salon must reach the target clients. Be sure to research the stations in your area before buying radio advertisement. The advertisement should include your specialty, the services you offer. Many radio advertisements for salons do not specify the chief product or service being advertised. Generally, the advertisements tell where the salon is located.

Advertising in this form really does not help the client decide whether to visit your establishment, so be specific. The salon owner needs to decide on the time needed for advertisement and the days of the week the advertisement will be run. For example, the salon owner should decide if a 30-second, 60-second, or musical piece for a period is sufficient. The salon owner will decide if the announcement will be made early in the morning, midday, or in the evening, as people drive home from work. All these elements are important to the success of your salon.

In television advertising, advertising is authentic. The advertisement can consist of dramatization of salon owner and staff. There can be small skits and other dramatized situations that represent the services being advertised. Commercials can be very "catchy" with the right people and the right sound effects. Most people remember a favorite commercial. Salon advertising has to be the same. The specialty salons have the opportunities to show their specialties. If a weave technique is being done on a client with healthy hair, the client may not mind if she is shown on the commercial. If a client is wearing a fashionable wig, she may not mind if she is included in the commercial. Most clients will do whatever they can for their stylist, if they are pleased with the stylist.

The advertisement should:

- Promote the overall beauty business
- Promote the specialty salon

- Tell the specific services being offered
- Tell the location of the salon and any landmarks near the salon
- Tell the telephone number of the salon
- Promote the prestige of the salon owner and staff
- Tell about new promotions and retail items
- Tell about any specials

In advertising, be sure the radio and/or television salesperson understands exactly what you want. Communication breakdowns can occur when discussing advertisement. Salon owners can become upset because they do not feel that they received what they asked for when purchasing the advertisement. For the best results, preview the advertisement. Make all changes at this time. For example, the salon owner might list prices. After listening on the radio or seeing how it looks on television, salon owners can change their minds. This is understandable, because everyone wants the services for which they are paying.

Business cards and flyers are other avenues to take to advertising. Some stylists and wig specialists seem shy when it comes to talking to people, some are afraid of rejection. Rejection erodes self-esteem. Being aggressive is a must in the beauty industry. Being overaggressive can be a problem for many clients, however. Clients do not seem to like people who appear "too pushy." Stylists who are too aggressive force clients away from them. Different people believe different things. Some say aggressiveness works; others say it is not necessary. Whether aggressive or passive, skills are still required to be a success in the beauty industry. Advertisement is a necessity for anyone who plans to have a career in the beauty industry. Newspapers are an option for the more passive stylist. A picture of the stylist can be on display in the newspaper, followed by all the special services the stylist offers. However the stylist plans to advertise, it is an individual, though necessary, choice.

Building Business Using the Computer and Telephone

The telephone and the computer are the main sources of reaching clients. Clients who listen to the radio or watch television will more than likely answer a telephone. If they do not answer a telephone, they will more than likely use a computer. Today, everything a person seems to need is on the computer. Specialty salons and general salons can use the computer to set up advertisement. The computer can be used as a vehicle to tell about the stylist or wig specialist. If stylists or wig specialists want to display their work, it can be done on the computer. For example, the author has a Web site promoting herself and her work (*www.tonilove.com*). Through the Web, the stylist can communicate with the world. The stylist can use the Web site to seek future business and clients.

The computer, if properly used, can really aid in the salon business. The salon can keep a list of clients. The list can include new clients, transient/walk-in clients, standing clients, and request clients. The main list of clients can allow the salon owner to evaluate the volume of business of the salon. The inventory of the salon can be kept. If the salon is a specialty salon, the salon owner wants to be sure to have all needed implements and supplies. The bills of the salon and the budget can be kept on the computer. If the budget is kept on computer files, every time money is depleted from the budget, it can be traced.

More salons are using computers, and they can see the difference it is making in their businesses. Salon owners believe their jobs have been made much easier by computers. Retail sales can also be recorded using computers. Some salon owners are not convinced that computers are the answers to their problems, so they still do everything manually. With computers, e-mails can be sent to clients who enjoy using computers. E-mail allows clients to visit the salon to see what is new. Specials and promotions can be sent through e-mail. Clients can visit the salon's Web site to see upcoming events, such as hair shows. The salon can post newsletters to tell the clients the latest hair trends for the season and what type of community services the salon is participating in. For example, the wig specialty salon may do a community-service project involving nursing homes and hospitals. Staff may decide to make and donate wigs to patients who need them. If this community-service event is on the salon's Web site, it generates business for the salon.

However, there is still the telephone. It is estimated that more people talk on the telephone than use the computer. The telephones in salons are therefore very important in generating business. Through proper use, the telephone is the salon's tool to make a good first impression. In public relations, the telephone and the person who answers it go hand in hand. The person must be compassionate, courteous, and friendly. All these traits must be heard in the voice of the receptionist. The person's voice must "smile" and make the client "smile." Therefore, clients will want to come to the salon, sometimes just to meet the person they were speaking with on the telephone.

Many salons do not make good first impressions, and clients are skeptical about visiting. Some clients do not visit after calling. Some clients interviewed said, "My day was going good until I called the salon," "That salon needs to replace that receptionist," "The receptionist acts as if she owns the salon, she's so rude on the telephone." If these remarks sound familiar, the following questions will help the salon owner reevaluate the situation:

- Does the phone ring more than twice before answering?
- Do the receptionists identify themselves?
- Does the receptionist talk when his or her mouth is full?
- Does the receptionist speak clearly?
- Does the receptionist try to sound friendly?
- Does the receptionist put clients on hold for long periods?
- Does the receptionist offer to take a message?
- Is the person answering the phone helpful?
- Does the receptionist obtain accurate information when taking messages?
- Does the receptionist go "the extra mile" in regards to manners?
- Does the receptionist say, "Thank You," when necessary?

When selecting a receptionist for the salon, the salon owner should make sure these traits are evident:

- Skilled in area
- Represents the image of the salon
- Well-groomed
- Experienced in public relations
- Computer literate
- Nice telephone voice
- Pleasing personality

These traits in the receptionist will lead to satisfied clients and an increase in business.

Displaying in Specialty Salons

Displays can stop potential clients in their tracks. Modern salons have displays that are very intricate. The windows of salons are adorned with mannequins and other décor to make the salons speak to the potential client. The salon seems to say, "Come in here," and the potential clients seem unable to resist. The display makes the potential client want a closer look. The display should be informative, yet leave something to the imagination.

Many salons have done away with displays. Others need displays to survive. Displays can be an asset, because they can place salons in classes of their own. In shopping for a location, many salon owners do not think as much about display area as they do the salon interior. Salon displays should tell a story. During Christmas and other holidays, many department stores use beautiful displays just to draw people to their store. Some displays are so popular, people travel all over the world just to see them.

Displays should reflect the personality of the salon and make clients feel at home. It is always a good idea to feature the most popular aspect of the salon. Wigs can come in many colors, as can hairpieces. Therefore, it is a smart retail and recruitment move to tell a colorful story using wigs and hairpieces. Some salons tie in local events such as high school homecoming themes, prom themes, and other local affiliations. If this is done, it makes the people involved in the community feel a part of the salon.

Lighting also plays an important role in displaying. Everything on display needs to be seen. Spotlights are very helpful in focusing on the main item to be promoted. At night, as people are passing by the salon, the light will usually make them stop. If the display is attractive enough, it will make them visit the salon. Displays using various arrays of color seem to be most popular. They create different feelings. Color is attractive to children. Children may insist to be brought to the salon for closer looks. If this happens, use communication and public relations skills to new recruit clients. It is up to the stylist to make prospective clients and real clients.

Though displays draw clients to a salon, the salon owner must make sure the displays are not overdone. Too much decoration can make the display look bad. If a display looks bad, it discourages clients. Clients may come, but to see the "bad-looking" display. Displays are not for everyone. They are less popular in salons that employ independent contractors as staff members. This is because the stylist or wig specialist is there only to rent the booth and the salon owner or receptionist has to attend to the displays.

Being a Salon Owner

Many people feel they have the attributes to be salon owners. This is not true. To be a successful salon owner, one thing is evident: The person has to be a leader. Not all people are able to lead, though some people feel they were born to lead. The leader of any establishment will agree that it is not always easy. Many salon owners feel it is one of the hardest jobs in existence. People who are leaders are subjected to all types of ridicule and disgruntled following. Many people shed the "limelight" of leadership just to keep peace of mind. Salon owners must concentrate on handling staff members and the problems that occur.

When handling people, the salon owner or manager must use tact and diplomacy, yet be assertive. It also helps if the owner knows how to compromise when necessary. The ability to teach follows. If a staff member feels the owner or manager has something to offer, or something that will be beneficial, the staff members will follow. If salon managers cannot cut or style hair or lack managerial skills, they will have problems.

Discipline is another trait of a good salon owner and manager. Discipline shown through the owner and manager helps the staff become self-disciplined. Leaders or salon owners and managers must lead by example. "Say what you mean and mean what you say," said one stylist.

The staff look to the manager for answers, because the owner is often not seen. The owner and manager need to inspire the staff. If the salon owner and manager have the ability to inspire, the most unmotivated staff members will feel like they need to do something. If a staff member shows self-motivation and initiative, the staff member should be rewarded. To be a successful salon owner and manager, the person must do the following, according to author Stewart Harral:

- Be fair.
- Be considerate.
- Be consistent.
- Use authority wisely.
- Use authority democratically.
- Stand behind principle.
- Possess sound judgment.
- Possess sound common sense.
- Possess emotional stability.
- Have a good sense of humor.
- Possess a high degree of social intelligence.
- Possess the drive to work hard.
- Possess the drive to work persistently.
- Learn the secret of getting the cooperation of others.
- Seek self-improvement.
- Set examples pertaining to conduct, methods, and goals.
- Possess an abiding faith in the worth of your profession.
- Be alert.
- Keep up with current events.
- Learn the concepts of public relations.

According to Forbes Magazine, there are the following:

- Five most important words: "I am proud of you."
- Four most important words: "What is your opinion?"
- Three most important words: "If you please."
- Two most important words: "Thank you."
- Least important word. "I."

Once a salon owner and manager learn and practice these traits, their salon will be a success.

Grievances in the Specialty Salon

In performing weaving and wig care, stylists are prone to having more grievances than general salons, some stylists argue, because clients are recreating themselves. As long as people think, opinions will differ. As a professional in the industry, one stylist said she learned a long time ago not to argue with a client. When a client has a complaint, the stylist should still have a smile. Some stylists take complaints personally. The legitimate complaint is rarely a personal attack. The stylist or wig specialist needs to understand that clients have rights, too. Stylists are not magicians, and they are not perfect. The stylist will not get everything right all the time.

Tact and discipline must be the forerunners of the stylist's or wig specialist's reactions. Sometimes, however, this is not the situation. The "dictatorial method" should not be used to handle grievances. Harral recommends the following procedure for handling grievances:

- Listen sympathetically—let the client speak.
- Get all the facts—not one side of the story.
- Look for the story behind the story.
- Make, or get, a decision.
- Sell your solution.
- Follow up—make sure promises are kept.
- Treat the other person as you would like to be treated.

The author also suggests the following to reduce the number of grievances:

- Know your clients.
- Take care of little things.
- Pay special attention to the differences in people.
- Be liberal with praise.
- Do not employ a disgruntled person.
- Watch for any situation that may produce a grievance.

After the salon owner and manager learn how to handle grievances properly, they can teach the salon staff. Once everyone has learned, the business will benefit.

Recruiting Salon Staff

If having the best salon is a dream, this portion of the chapter is crucial. Recruiting is popular in schools, salons, and other businesses. Everyone is looking for the "best" employee. The life of the salon depends heavily on who is working *with* you. A lot of people use the word *for*, but when people come into your establishment, make them feel a part of the establishment.

The newly employed person would love to hear an owner or manager express that they are working with them to make the salon a better place to work. There are several methods of recruiting. Some salon owners and managers circulate posters among the beauty salons in their areas. Advertisements are placed in the newspaper, on the radio, and on television. High schools have become primary targets, because a lot of the high schools teach cosmetology. Young students can be trained for longevity. Advertising in professional journals and magazines has become a pretty popular method of recruiting. Showcasing is done for activities of the salon, such as hair shows, hair-cutting drives for a special cause, or a community-service project. These activities often help in recruiting, because everyone wants to be a part of the "winning team." If it seems as if your salon is productive and positive, people will come to you. Another recruiting tool is establishing scholarships, high school and college. A "school-to-work" program between a school and your salon would really aid in recruiting. Students will have the opportunity to work before completing school, and the salon owner and manager can observe. Do not become a "nuisance" and start bothering people about working for you. If you call prospective employees too much, more than likely you will scare them away. If the salon owner or manager have "first emotions" that seem negative about a prospective employee, the salon owner or manager should trust those feelings.

If salon owners or managers feel that a person is right, in most cases they are right. Many people make the mistake of not checking references. Always check references. Because recruiting can be frustrating, a lot of salon owners fill their salons with people they do not like or people with whom they are not satisfied. Keep the details of recruiting for your salon simple and clear. As poet Maya Angelou said, "When people show you who they are, believe them."

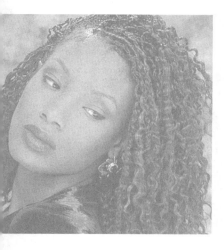

Safety Precautions

- Always consult with clients.
- Always do a hair and scalp analysis.
- Be sure you understand what clients are asking before performing services.
- Learn weave techniques before performing them.
- Never pull or tug the thread while weaving.
- During fusion, never allow the hot adhesive to touch the skin.
- In making wigs, always keep the wefts close together.
- Always protect the clients.
- Use the proper capes for services.
- Always recheck wig measurements.
- In cutting wigs, never lose the guideline.
- Thin wigs with thinning shears for best results.
- Always wear gloves when performing chemical services.

- Be sure rubberbands used for weaving are not tight.
- Be sure braids are not tight.
- When doing extensions, be sure the hair is not too heavy.
- When locking the hair, be sure to use correct "locking" supplies.
- Do not use excessive heat on synthetic hair.
- If unsure about the type of commercial hair, always do the "match test."
- Always analyze skin type before applying commercial hair.
- Always check facial type before making hairstyle recommendations.
- Be sure wigs fit securely.
- Be sure clients select colors that are complementary to their skin types and lifestyles.
- If clients wear glasses, consider them when styling.
- Be consistent in prices.
- Take great care when combing or brushing wigs to avoid matting.
- When cleaning a wig or hairpiece, never rub or wring out the fluid.
- When you shape (cut) a wig or hairpiece, use great care. Once the hair has been cut, it cannot grow back.
- When you comb a freshly set wig, use a wide-tooth comb to help you gain greater control and to avoid damaging the wig's foundation.
- When you clean or work with a wet wig, always mount it on a block of the same head size as the wig to avoid stretching.
- Take accurate measurements of the client's head to ensure a comfortable and secure fit.
- Recondition wigs as often as needed to prevent dry or brittle hair.
- If needed, clean wigs before setting and styling.
- Brush and comb wigs and hairpieces with a downward movement.
- Never lighten (bleach) a wig or hairpiece.
- Never give a permanent to a wig or hairpiece.

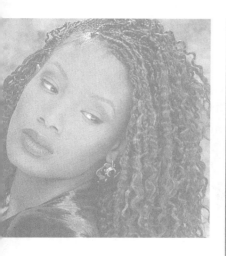

Glossary

Asian/European hair—Very straight hair.

Commercial hair—Hair applied to natural hair for styling purposes.

Consultation—Meeting between the stylist or wig specialist and the client. Held before any hair services are performed.

Dreadlocks—Hair that is twisted and allowed to grow in twisted formation.

Excess weight—Hair that is too heavy and thick.

Fill-ins—Hair covering areas of thinning extensions.

Foundation—Solid base for weave formation. Results from braiding or interlocking.

Fusion—Hair-extension technique using an adhesive available in different colors.

Growth—Natural hair extending from the scalp.

Hair extensions—Extension of natural hair using commercial hair and various techniques.

Hair matting—When the hair is tangled.

Hairpiece—Commercial hair that is not on a weft. Can be added to specific areas.

Hair repairs—Commercial hair of the weave needs tightening or the wig needs reconditioning.

Hair shaping—Cutting the hair into a style.

Infusion—Hair-extension technique using bonding glue available in different colors.

Natural hair—The client's own hair. May be referred to as "virgin" hair.

New growth—Growth of chemically relaxed hair. New (virgin) hair that has grown after chemical relaxer was applied.

Price list—List of all salon services and their prices.

Shears—Scissors.

Synthetic hair—Hair made from synthetic fibers or kanekalon.

Thinning shears—Scissors used to thin hair and reduce bulk.

Toupee—Commercial hair worn mostly by men. Available in human hair or synthetic fiber.

Underlaying—Placing commercial hair under natural hair or another section of commercial hair.

Weave—Process of placing commercial hair on natural hair until the two are blended for styling.

Weaving needles—Tools for weaving techniques. Available straight, curved, or straight with curved tips.

Weaving pole—Mostly wooden pole used to aid the hair weaver. Usually secures the weaving thread and decreases thread tangling.

Weaving thread—Thread used to perform weaving techniques with the needle. Comes in different colors.

Wig coloring—Applying permanent color, semipermanent color, or temporary color to a human-hair wig.

Yak hair—Commercial hair that is close in texture to overcurly hair.

Index